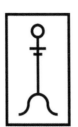

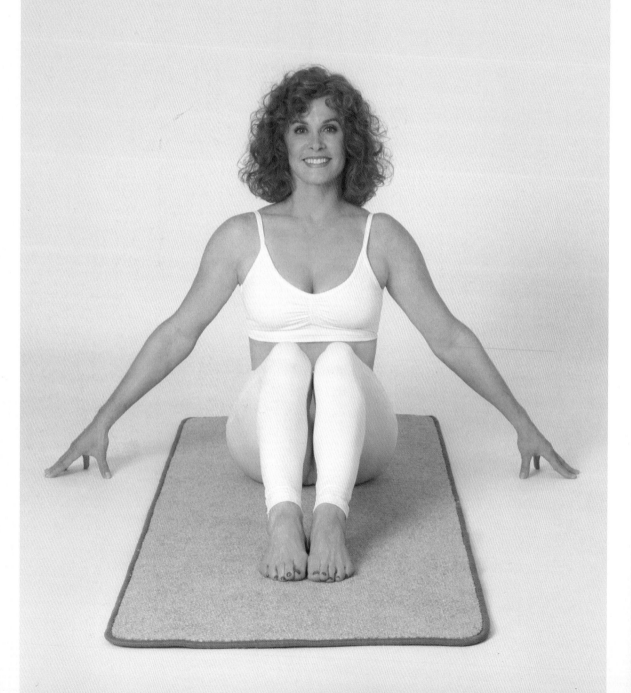

POWERS
PILATES

STEFANIE POWERS' GUIDE TO LONGEVITY AND WELL-BEING THROUGH PILATES

STEFANIE POWERS

AND
KATHY COREY
MASTER TEACHER

A FIRESIDE BOOK
PUBLISHED BY SIMON & SCHUSTER
NEW YORK   LONDON   TORONTO   SYDNEY

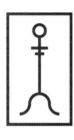

FIRESIDE
Rockefeller Center
1230 Avenue of the Americas
New York, NY 10020

FIRESIDE and colophon are registered trademarks
of Simon & Schuster, Inc.

For information regarding special discounts for bulk purchases,
please contact Simon & Schuster Special Sales at 1-800-456-6798 or
business@simonandschuster.com

Designed by Bridget Morley

Manufactured in China
10 9 8 7 6 5 4 3 2 1

Library of Congress Cataloging-in-Publication data is available

ISBN 0-7432-5627-1

CAUTION
The techniques, ideas, and suggestions in this book are to be used at
the reader's sole discretion and risk. Always follow the instructions
carefully, observe the cautions, and consult a doctor if in doubt about a
medical condition.

I can never forget that old joke about the man who reaches a grand old age and says, "if I knew I was going to live this long, I would have taken better care of myself"...

STEFANIE POWERS

Contents

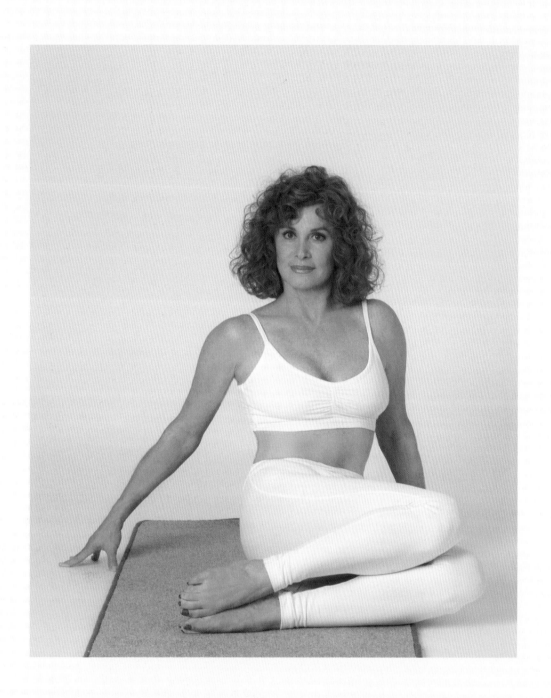

INTRODUCTION

It is a fact that we actually do have the potential of living far longer lives than even our parents' generation. Knowing this is true, it is entirely up to us to choose how we might prepare ourselves to enjoy that possibility.

I began my career as a dancer and, while working with Jerome Robbins and his New York-based dancers, I heard people refer to the wonders of Joseph Pilates' techniques and how they helped dancers who were injured while performing. Some years later when I was in New York, I happened to pass the Pilates studio on 57th Street, so I couldn't help but take a peek. What I saw was incomprehensible: strange-looking handles dangling from springs and odd apparatus. I didn't stay long enough to talk to anyone.

Some years later, a friend told me about a wonderful class given by a former Martha Graham dancer called Ron Fletcher. Lots of actors I knew were getting in shape for work with his help, so I went and discovered a world and a philosophy of well-being that has remained with me ever since.

One of Ron's disciples, Kathy Corey, expresses Joseph Pilates' technique in this way:

It is the mind itself which shapes the body.

It is the breath that feels the movement.

It is the union of these elements that uplifts the spirit and promotes well-being.

Body, Mind, & Spirit.

Kathy is now a master teacher and has played a major part in designing the program in this book.

I believe strongly that internalizing exercise improves the body and mind and helps us feel as if we are inside our body and not just using it as motive power.

Longevity and well-being are a desirable state, but one without the other does not encourage a good quality of life.

Like the old man who wished he had taken better care of himself, we now have the tools and the method to do just that, and in so doing, extend our ability to get the most out of our longer lives.

ABOUT THE PILATES METHOD

Joseph Pilates was born in Germany in 1880 and died in New York City in 1967. As a child, he was sickly and frail but was determined to overcome his disadvantages. By the time he was 14 and after extensive gymnastic training, young Joseph was posing for photographs for anatomy charts.

During World War I, Joseph Pilates was interned in England and worked as a nurse with injured soldiers, applying his methods of physical training as therapy. The results were amazing. Pilates' patients recovered noticeably faster and in better shape than those he had not treated. After the war, it was his collaboration with Rudolph von Laban that exposed Pilates to the world of dance.

In 1926, Joseph Pilates set up his first studio in New York City and attracted interest among the legendary dancers and choreographers of the day, including Martha Graham and George Balanchine. Pilates' studio soon became a magnet for dancers of all disciplines who sought help with conditioning and recovery.

POWERS ON PILATES

I think it is useful to imagine that your body is nothing but a bag of bones – 206 bones to be precise – supported by ligaments, tendons, and 639 muscles. This is our support system. It keeps us upright and defies gravity. Over time and without proper bodywork, it is gravity that causes us to collapse in the center, to bend, and literally shrink. Joseph Pilates' technique is not a traditional exercise program, it is a way of life. It helps us to perform our daily activities with increased consciousness and, above all, balance and support.

Why should balance and support be so important? Because proper alignment, supported by good muscle tone, helps to keep our organs in place and keep at bay the negative results of a weakened and lop-sided framework.

One of the greatest components of Pilates' bodywork is the breathing. For centuries, yogis have understood the benefits of proper breathing to the entire cardiovascular system. In our hectic lives we pay little attention to taking a breath and, in so doing, slowly starve ourselves of oxygen. It is our circulatory system that suffers most.

This book is a reflection of classical Pilates' movement patterns to improve flexibility, posture, and alignment. Above all, they create deep core strength without stressing the joints or adding bulk to the body.

The only props enlisted in developing this program are a towel, a chair, and a floor mat. The movement sequence has been carefully designed to encourage alignment, while toning and stretching the entire body.

Joseph Pilates was far ahead of his time, but fortunately his work has been passed on to the benefit of us all.

It is true that the only good exercise is the one you do – so let's begin!

1 The basics

* ## Alignment and centering

* ## Core balance

* ## Breathing

Alignment and centering

All movement originates in the torso, which is the strength center of the body, and the pelvic girdle, which supports the spine. As time passes, gravity causes the vertebrae to press down on each other. The weight of the head, rounded shoulders, and poor posture add to the problem, increasing curvature in the shoulder and waist areas.

To benefit fully from the Pilates method your spine, head, and pelvic girdle need to be correctly aligned. You also need to direct your concentration inside your body. This centering increases your awareness of your organs and systems, restoring the connection between body and mind.

Many of the exercises in this program start with this alignment and centering, a combination we call "the starting position".

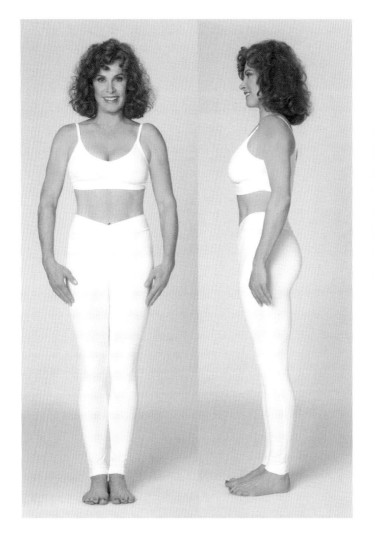

What you should feel
Your spine feels longer, as if you are growing taller. The pressure in your lower back releases and your chest feels open.

1 Stand with your knees and ankles together. Hold your shoulders back and down so they are relaxed. Raise your chin a little and let your arms hang at your sides, with your hands loose. Make sure your knees are not locked.

2 Without tucking your pelvis under, squeeze your buttocks as tight as you can. Lift upward and inward with your stomach muscles.

3 Pull your stomach in and up, as if you were lifting up and off your hips. Keep your shoulders down. Feel yourself almost separate your torso from your pelvic girdle.

4 Elongate the bones in the back of your neck, causing the back of the jaw to release.

Core balance

Core balance works in harmony with alignment as the foundation and base of the body. Using your feet as a platform to support your aligned body, feel yourself connecting with gravity. Make sure that your weight is evenly distributed between both feet. We often lean forward too much, destroying our alignment.

It may help to visualize a triangle on the sole of each foot. The triangle links your big toe, little toe, and the center of your heel.

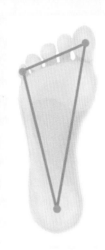

Don't
* lift your chin up too high
* arch your back
* lock your knees
* lift your shoulders
* lean forward
* tense your toes

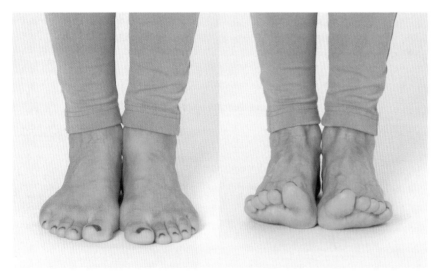

1 *Stand in the alignment position (see Step 1, p.13), with your feet together.*

2 *Lift up your toes and evenly distribute your weight into the*

triangle. Your posture naturally tilts very slightly backward.

3 *Lower your toes. Now you are in alignment.*

Breathing

The technique of breathing has a sound and a rhythmical pattern. It enhances lung capacity and improves the oxygenation of red blood cells. You will feel the difference and easily focus on the exercise. (See also Advanced breathing, pp.128-29.)

This technique is a major part of every exercise, although the number of counts will vary.

Audibly suck in air through your nose to a mental count of, for example, five. Then breathe out through your mouth to the same count, with a shushing sound. Make the breaths into short, rhythmic bursts — in, in, in, in, in and shush, shush, shush, shush, shush — and pace them to the counting inside your head.

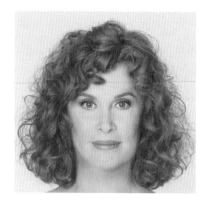

I *Breathe in through your nose.*

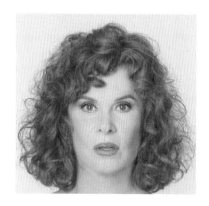

2 *Breathe out through your mouth with a shushing sound.*

Don't
* rush the breathing
* lose contact with your core alignment

What you should feel
You should feel slightly light-headed and a tingling throughout your body

Now you are ready to start!

2 Warm-ups

* Single foot rolls

* Foot rolls with press

* Toe lifts

* Core balance

* Half-circle neck stretch

* Cross-foot stretch

* Finger flicks

No matter what time of day, either morning or afternoon, warm-up stretches help to loosen tight muscles and circulate the blood, waking up the connective tissue and enhancing flexibility. Simply put, the more you stretch the more you will be able to extend the stretch. This fact is particularly important for our feet because, even though we spend plenty of time walking or standing, they are the least exercised part of the body. Perhaps we feel that our feet don't need exercise because they get enough! When you begin to exercise your feet, you will soon realize their general lack of flexibility. The same is true for our hands and fingers.

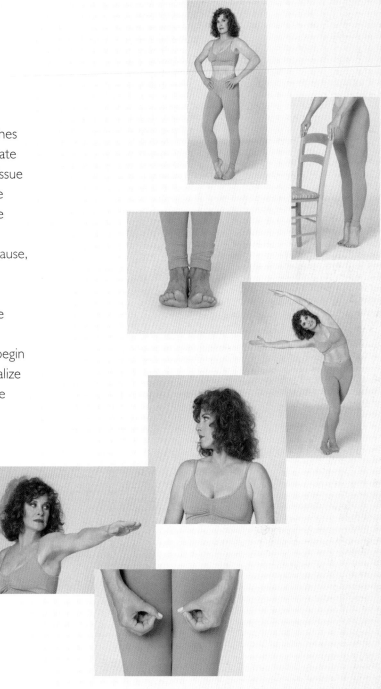

Single foot rolls

Just as a tree is only as strong as its roots, the body depends on the feet as its support base or platform.

Do this exercise in front of a mirror and look carefully at how raising a heel can affect your entire body.

Breathing pattern

• Inhale for a count of four as you raise your heel from the floor.

• Exhale for a count of four as you lower your heel to the floor.

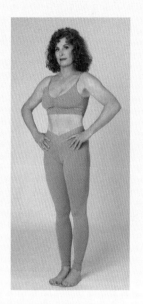

Starting position
Stand with your feet together, hands on hips, and your weight evenly distributed. Align your body (see p.13).

Do's and dont's
* Keep your knee centered over the front of your foot.
* Don't roll your foot inward or outward. * Don't lift or sway your hips as you roll up or down.

What you should feel
After a few repetitions you should feel a loosening in the toes and better circulation in your feet.

Repetitions
Repeat the exercise 16 times, alternating your feet.

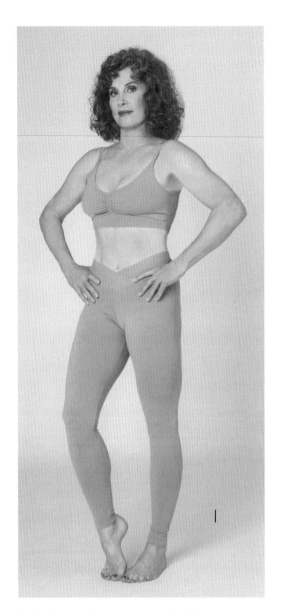

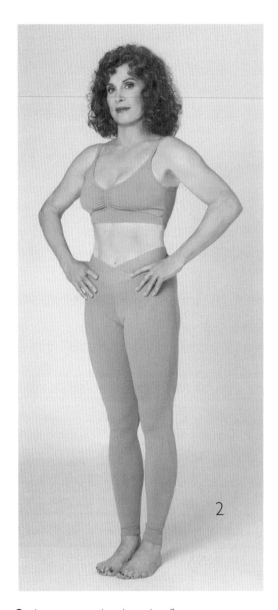

1 *Roll one foot on to the ball, keeping your body weight directly over the center of your foot.*

2 *Lower your heel to the floor.*

Variation
As you gain more mobility through your foot, hold up your heel for a count of ten, inhaling for five and exhaling for five.

Foot rolls with press

With age and lack of exercise, the muscles in the feet lose their strength and the arches begin to drop. If you practice this exercise three times a day, the blood flow to the feet will increase, eliminating the toxins that have accumulated due to poor circulation. You can do the exercise sitting down on long trips to help prevent your feet swelling.

Breathing pattern

• Inhale for a count of five as you raise your heel.

• Exhale for a count of five as you press.

• Inhale as you raise your heel.

• Exhale as you lower your foot.

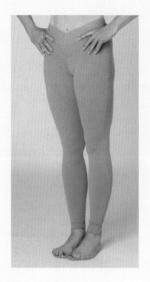

Starting position
Stand or sit with your feet together and align your body (see p.13).

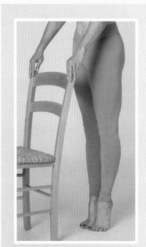

Variation
For a more advanced movement, hold on to the back of a chair or wall for balance and practice the exercise while raising both heels at the same time.

Repetitions
Repeat the exercise 16 times, alternating your feet.

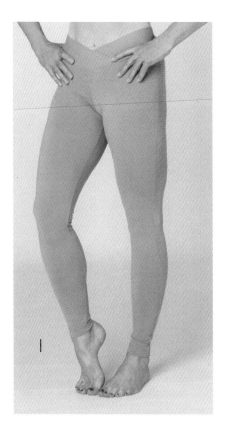

I *Roll on to the furthest point on the ball of your foot, pressing your body weight into it. Do not twist your foot or sway your body – simply keep your posture aligned, placing even pressure across the foot, from the big to the little toe.*

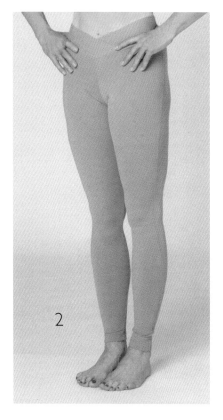

2 *Lower your heel to the floor.*

What you should feel
Your toes, especially the big toe, should feel increasingly flexible. As you press further forward on the ball of your foot there will be an increased circulation of blood.

Toe lifts

You will be amazed at the amount of strength in your toes and how much they are used to balance your body. This movement strengthens the muscles on the top of your feet and increases the flow of blood into your toes. Cold feet and poor circulation can lead to stiff, painful feet and cause problems that affect the rest of your body.

Breathing pattern

• Inhale for a count of two as you lift up your toes.

• Exhale for a count of two as you lower your toes to the floor.

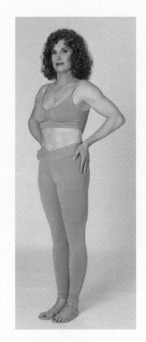

Starting position
Stand with your feet together and align your body (see p.13).

Variation
Try the exercise using one foot at a time. Then try it while lowering each toe, one at a time.

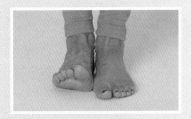 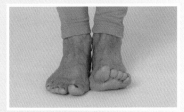

Repetitions
Repeat the exercise ten times.

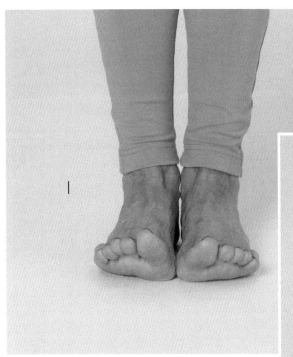

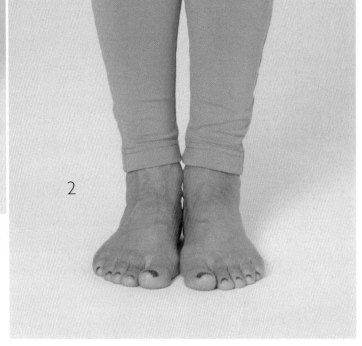

I *Lift up the toes of both feet, pressing the bones (metatarsals) at the base of your toes strongly and evenly into the floor. Do not roll your feet inward or outward, and do not lean back as you lift.*

2 *Lower your toes to the floor, stretching them apart and placing each toe firmly down.*

Core balance

To test that you are aligned physically and centered mentally, try doing the toe lifts with your eyes closed. Feel yourself coming into balance from the inside of your body outward.

Breathing pattern

• Inhale as you lift your toes.

• Exhale as you close your eyes.

• Breath deeply, inhaling and exhaling with your eyes closed.

• Inhale and open your eyes, and exhale as you lower your toes.

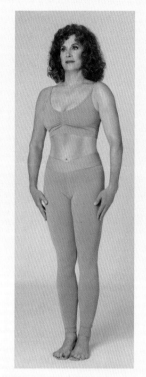

Starting position
Align your body and find your center (see p.13).

Do's and dont's
* Don't roll your foot inward or outward. * Keep your knee centred over the front of your foot. * Do not lift or sway your hips as you roll up or down.

Variations
Practice this exercise at the end of the program to feel how just one session has made you more centered and aligned.

As you become more stable from your core, add another breath with your eyes closed. Work up to five breaths with your eyes closed and toes lifted.

Repetitions
Repeat the exercise five times.

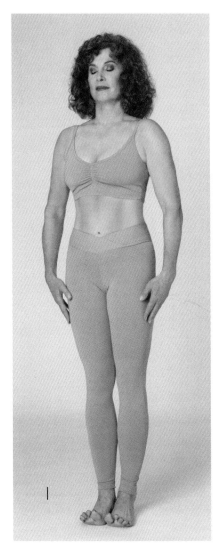

1 Close your eyes. Inhale and exhale deeply. Then inhale as you lift your toes.

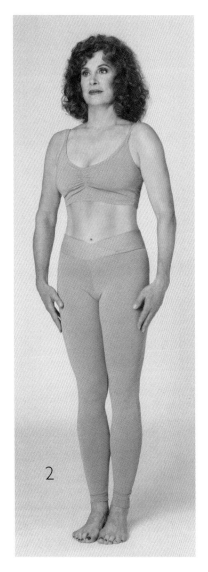

2 *Open your eyes and exhale as you lower your toes.*

What you should feel
At first, you may feel disorientated. If you focus your mind on your center within you, you may start to feel the freedom of balance.

Half-circle neck stretch

This exercise lengthens the neck muscles to decrease stress and tension, which can cause constriction of blood vessels to the head and brain. It also improves the firmness of the muscles under the chin – definitely a good thing to do!

Breathing pattern

• Inhale for a count of two as you bring your chin to your chest.

• Exhale for a count of two as you rotate your head over your shoulder.

• Do the small pulses with two short inhalations and two short exhalations for a count of eight.

Variation
Add more pulses as your neck muscles strengthen.

Do's and don'ts
* Keep your shoulders directly over your hips.
* Don't hunch forward as you start the exercise.

Repetitions
Repeat the exercise four times.

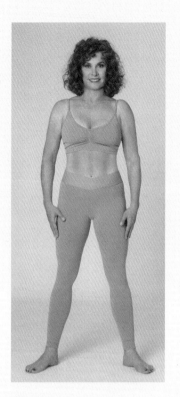

Starting position
Stand with your feet hip-distance apart. Relax your arms at your sides. Make sure your shoulders are directly over your hips.

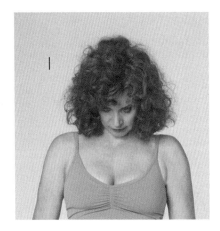

1 Lower your head, bringing your chin to your chest.

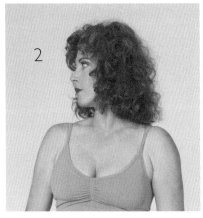

2 Circle your head over your shoulder, bringing your chin parallel to the floor while pressing your opposite shoulder down.

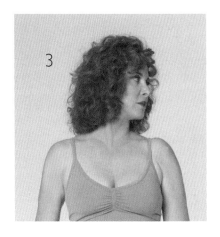

3 Slowly and gently rotate your chin to your chest again, lengthening your neck, while pulling your shoulders away from your ears. Circle your head to the opposite shoulder. Return your chin to your chest.

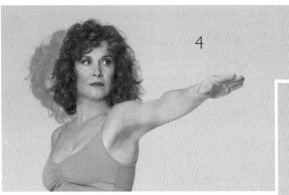

4 Circle your head over your shoulder, lifting one arm up to shoulder level.

5 Pulse your head over your shoulder with eight small pulses. Lower your arm and bring your chin to your chest. Repeat on the opposite side.

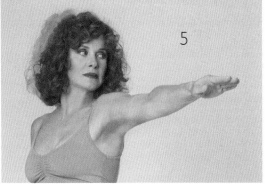

What you should feel
As the blood flow increases, the tension in the muscles of your neck and upper back should relax.

27

Cross-foot stretch

These side-bending movements stretch your torso and balance the trunk muscles on both sides of your body. These exercises also trim your waistline and improve your core stability.

Breathing pattern

• Inhale for a count of two and lift your arms over your head, keeping your shoulders back and down, and your chin in alignment.

• Exhale for a count of two as you lift and cross your foot, balancing on the ball of the foot.

• Inhale for a count of two as you lift and stretch over. Exhale to a count of two as you begin to reach the maximum stretch.

• Inhale for a count of two as you lift up to the center. Exhale at the center to a count of two.

• At the maximum stretch, exhale once at each of the eight pulses.

Do's and dont's
* Keep a very tight support from the squeezed muscles of your buttocks and tightened stomach.
* Never release this support during the entire exercise.
* Balance your body weight equally on both feet to create a stable support base for your stretch.
* Stretch directly to the side, keeping your hips and shoulders in a straight line. * Don't bend forward.
* Stretch as far as is comfortable for you.

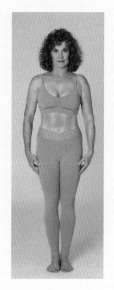

Starting position
Stand with your feet together. Align your body with your weight equally on both feet.

Variations
If you cannot balance with your arms over your head, hold them out to the side at shoulder level or place your fingertips lightly on a chair for balance.

When you can do the exercise with core stability, hold your foot in the air for a count of ten before returning it to the floor.

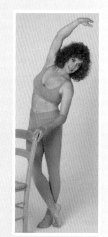

Repetitions
Repeat the whole exercise four times.

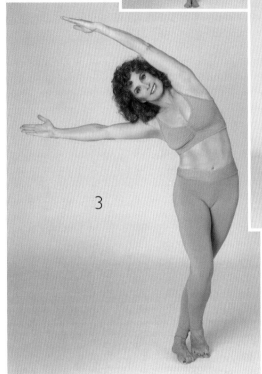

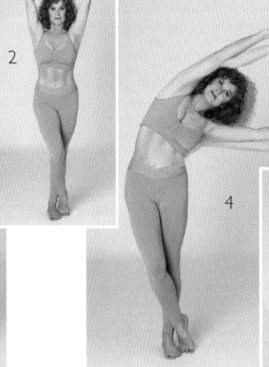

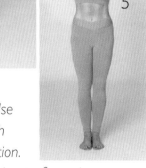

1 *Hold out your arms at shoulder level.*

2 *Lift your arms over your head. Roll to the ball of one foot. Maintain your alignment as you lift this foot off the floor, across your other foot, and place the ball of the foot on the floor.*

3 *Stretch up, over, and away from your crossed foot. Feel as if you are reaching for the ceiling and the walls.*

Repeat this stretch four times, alternating sides.

4 *Now repeat the stretch, adding a pulsing motion. Pulse eight times, exhaling at each pulse on the downward motion. Pulse your torso over, stretching as far as is comfortable with small movements.*

5 *Change sides and repeat the eight pulses.*

Finger flicks

This exercise improves the circulation in your arms and hands. The increased blood flow into the fingertips helps to flush out toxins and may reduce arthritis in the joints. The exercise also strengthens the muscles in the forearms and is excellent for alleviating tennis elbow.

Breathing pattern

Match your breath to the finger flicks by inhaling for two flicks, then exhaling for the next two flicks. Keeping this pattern throughout the cycle may be difficult at first, but it will become easier with practice.

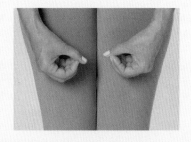

Starting position
Stand with your feet together. Bring your hands in front of you and make loose fists by rolling up your fingers with your thumb on top.

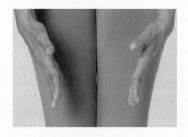

Flicking
Strongly flick your fingers open, as if you are trying to remove something sticky. You should hear a sound as your fingers stretch apart.

Variation
Once you have completed the cycle clockwise, switch the direction. Hold your arms out to the sides of your body and then over your head. Lower them in front of your body to complete the exercise.

What you should feel
Your wrists and forearms should feel lighter due to the increased blood flow.

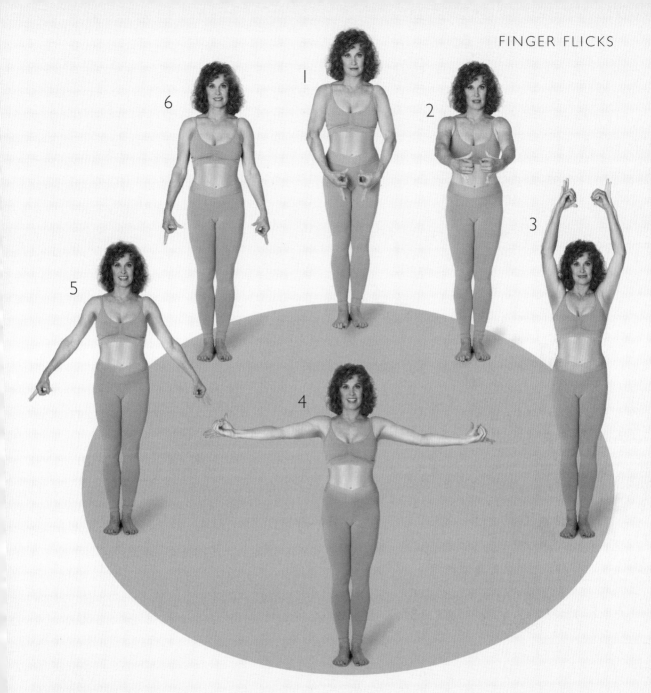

Flicking is continuous, even when you change position.

Do eight flicks while you stand in position 1 and four flicks as you move into position 2. Do eight flicks while standing in position 2 and four flicks as you move into position 3. Continue this pattern throughout the cycle.

Keep your wrists still so you can feel the exercise in your forearms as well as in your hands. The stronger your hand movement the more your forearms will benefit. Try to keep your arms straight in every position.

31

3 Towel work

* Towel lifts

* Taut pulls

* Towel pull-downs

* Chest pull-backs

* Overhead presses

* Backward stretch and lift

* Small presses up

* Arm, back, and chest stretch

* Side stretch

* Side stretch with cross arm

* Overhead twist

* Hip pulses

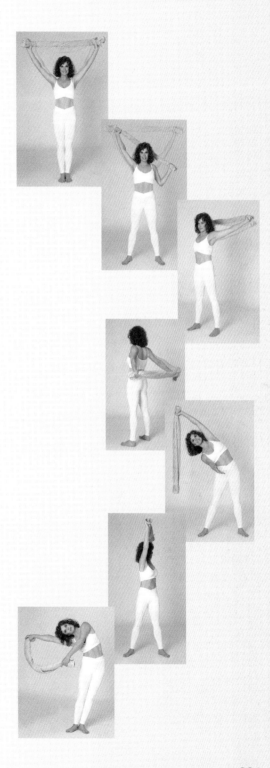

The towel used in the following exercises provides resistance for your muscles, making them work harder and strengthening your body. The towel needs to be soft yet sturdy and about 125cm (50in) long. Roll it up length-wise, then gently twist it. During the exercises, hold the ends of the towel lightly in your hands, without gripping tightly or bending your wrists. Keep your fingers relaxed.

Yoga bands, CORE bands, and thera-bands can work better than a towel since they are less likely to strain the muscles in the hands and do not untwist during the work.

As you lift the towel over your head, keep your shoulders down and maintain your alignment. Always lift the towel by engaging the muscles under your shoulder blades. This creates a support system through the muscle groups in your upper back, chest, shoulders, and neck that helps them become healthy and strong.

Overhead presses help to open your shoulders, while back stretches and lifts further improve flexibility. Presses up, stretches, twists, and pulses all add to your overall strength and flexibility, and aid in lubricating your joints.

Towel lifts

This exercise engages your shoulders, preparing them for activity and increasing the range of motion in your upper body. Lifting your arms over your head activates your chest and upper back muscles, which is vital for lifting and reaching movements. Keep pulling the towel taut and work slowly – and don't forget your core alignment.

Breathing pattern

- Inhale as you lift the towel to your chest.

- Exhale as you lift the towel over your head.

- Inhale as you bring the towel in front of your chest.

- Exhale as you lower your towel.

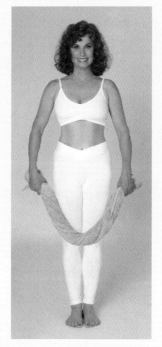

Starting position
Stand with your feet together, holding your towel lightly in front of you.

What you should feel
As your shoulder girdle opens, you should feel your shoulder joints becoming more flexible and your chest muscles opening, while your upper back strengthens.

Variations
If you release the core alignment in your upper torso, or start swaying as you lift the towel overhead, lift it only to chest level. With each repetition, lift it a little higher.

As the movement becomes easy, pull your shoulder blades down and in toward your spine for a count of five when you hold the towel overhead. Hold this position as you lower your towel to chest level and down.

Repetitions
Repeat this exercise ten times.

34

1 *Pull the towel taut and lift it to chest level.*

2 *Lift the towel over your head, keeping your ribcage in and your shoulders down. Don't sway or arch your back.*

3 *Lower the towel back to chest level.*

4 *Lower the towel down in front of your body.*

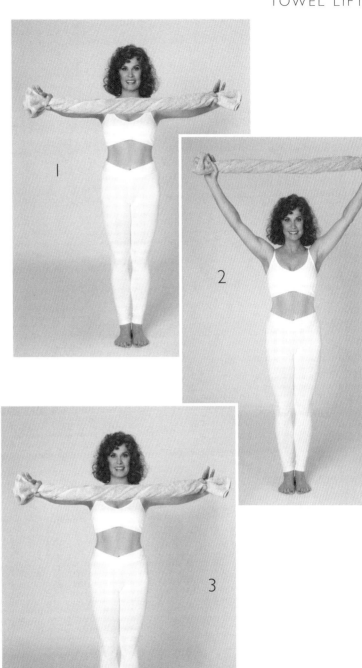

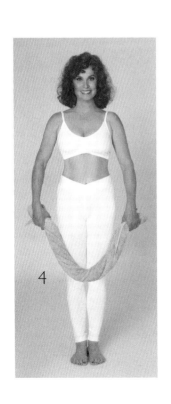

35

Taut pulls

This exercise helps to build a healthy back and spine. It activates your middle back muscles and stimulates the smaller, deeper muscles closer to your spine. It also increases the circulation to the connective tissues attached to your spine.

Breathing pattern

• Inhale for a count of four as you lift the towel over your head.

• Exhale as you pull the towel taut.

• Add a double inhale and a double exhale for a count of two on the small pulses.

• Take a full breath and lower the towel on an exhale.

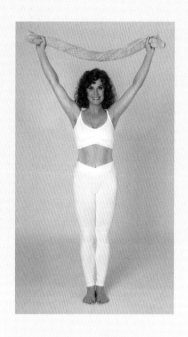

Starting position
Stand with your feet together and lift the towel over your head.

What you should feel
Your arms will become less tired as your back muscles do more work.

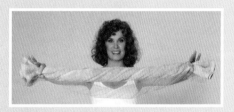

Variations
If you cannot lift your arms overhead, hold them in front of your chest. Keep your shoulders pulled back and down. You can also do the exercise sitting down.

As you progress, hold the towel taut for a count of five, with a long exhale. Take a long inhale as you release, and repeat.

Repetitions
Repeat this exercise three times.

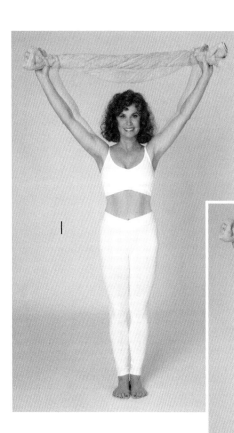

1 Pull the towel taut, keeping it directly over the center of your head. Release the pull, but keep the towel above your head.

Continue to pull and release four times.

2 Keep the towel over your head and pull it taut.

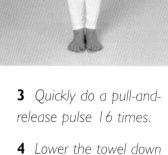

3 Quickly do a pull-and-release pulse 16 times.

4 Lower the towel down in front of your body.

Don't
* lift your shoulders
* lose the support of tightened buttock and stomach muscles

Towel pull-downs

This movement helps you to fight the pull of gravity and the forward slouch of your shoulders. It stretches your chest as it works deep into your back muscles.

Breathing pattern

• Inhale as you pull down the towel and exhale as you lift up, both for a count of two.

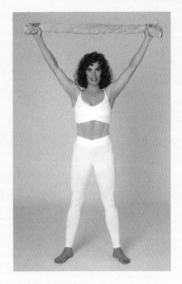

What you should feel
The tension and tight muscles in the upper torso will be released, increasing your flexibility. You will also feel a stretch from your chest to under each arm.

Starting position
Stand with your feet apart. Lift the towel over your head and pull it taut.

Do's and don'ts
* Hold your torso alignment and support. * Keep your shoulders lowered. * Don't let your head drop forward. * Don't release your hips or ribcage as you pull the towel down behind your head. * Don't arch your back.

Variation
Perform only as many movements and repeated steps as you can, but always maintain your core alignment. As your chest and back muscles start to work in balance, start to add repetitions to the exercise.

Repetitions
Do the sequence only once.

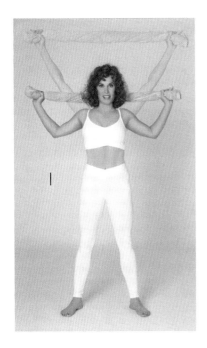

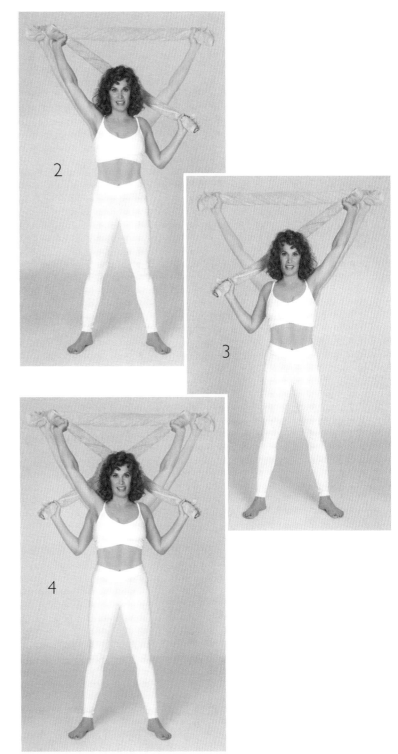

1 *Keep the towel taut as you pull it down behind your head to shoulder level, bending your arms. Pull your elbows down at the sides of your body, toward your waist. Lift the towel over your head, straightening your arms. Repeat this step eight times.*

2 *Keep one arm raised and pull the other down toward your waist. Return to the overhead position. Repeat this step four times.*

3 *Change arms and repeat Step 2.*

4 *Repeat the exercise eight times, alternating your arms.*

Complete the exercise by repeating the movement with both arms, four times.

Chest pull-backs

Throughout this exercise, you must maintain resistance to help you tone your torso muscles, thereby decreasing muscle exhaustion. As you press forward with your arms and resist with your stomach and entire torso, you build extra support for your back by strengthening the front. Your arms will not tire so that you can carry on holding up the towel.

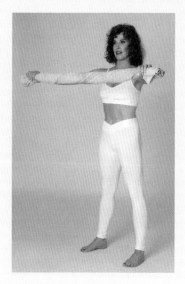

Breathing pattern

• Inhale for a count of two as you pull the towel toward you.

• Exhale for a count of two as you straighten your arms.

What you should feel
You should feel the muscles of your back, chest, and torso tighten and the blood circulate.

Starting position
Stand with your feet apart. Lift the towel to chest level and pull it taut. Activate your abdominal muscles and align your torso, pulling your ribcage in and down.

Do's and don'ts
* Keep your shoulder blades down and together.
* Keep your elbows shoulder-height throughout.
* Don't drop the height of the towel as you press forward. * Don't rotate your torso.

Variation
If you feel tension in your neck or shoulders, do fewer repetitions. Lower the towel, realign your torso and begin again.

As you progress, move more slowly. Count to four as you pull the towel to your chest and as you straighten your arms. Add a double inhale and double exhale to increase chest expansion and oxygenate the body.

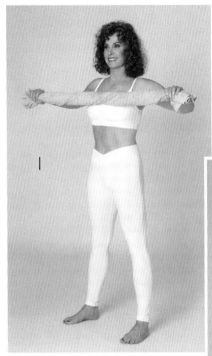

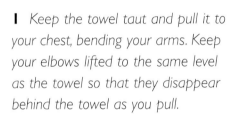

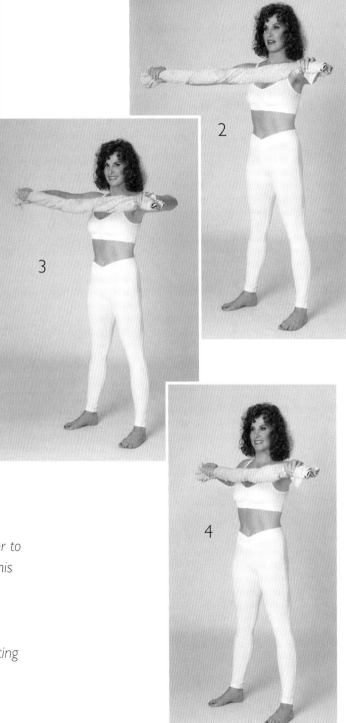

1 Keep the towel taut and pull it to your chest, bending your arms. Keep your elbows lifted to the same level as the towel so that they disappear behind the towel as you pull.

2 Straighten your arms, moving the taut towel out in front of you.

Repeat Steps 1 and 2 eight times.

3 Hold one arm out straight. Pull the other to your chest and then straighten it. Repeat this movement four times.

4 Change arms and repeat Step 3.

Repeat Steps 3 and 4 eight times, alternating your arms.

Complete the exercise by repeating the movement with both arms, four times.

Overhead presses

When your shoulders, chest, and upper back are open, the range of motion in your arms and upper torso increases in a very short time. At first, you may need to shorten your range of motion in order to work on opening your shoulders. If you press through the progression of the positions in this exercise and lose your alignment or lift your shoulders, you will not develop the ability to increase your stretch.

Breathing pattern

• Take a full breath in and out as you lift the towel over your head and realign your torso before starting the pulses.

• Use a double inhale and double exhale breathing pattern for each of the pulses.

• Inhale as you lift the towel over your head. Exhale as you bend your knees and lower the towel.

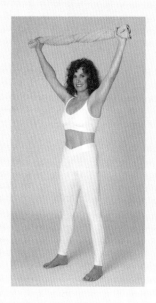

Starting position
Stand with your feet apart. Bring your arms over your head, pulling the towel taut. Pull down your shoulders and shoulder blades in order to stabilize them.

What you should feel
The mobility of your shoulders will increase as you stretch your back, chest, and upper torso. You will feel a tightness in your upper back and your circulation will increase.

Variation
Once the shoulder girdle has achieved full rotation, hold the towel in your most advanced position and bend your elbows until the towel touches your back between your shoulder blades. Straighten your arms behind your back, without locking your elbows. Repeat this movement four times before lifting the towel over your head.

1 *Keep your arms straight and bring them behind your head. Pulse backward, with eight small pulses, until the towel reaches behind the center of your head.*

2 *Bring the towel forward over your head. Bring your arms down and bend your knees. Straighten your legs and lift the towel over your head again.*

3 *Rotate your arms further behind your head, beginning the exercise where you ended your last set. Pulse back eight times.*

4 *Bring your arms overhead, bend your knees, and lower your arms down. Straighten your legs and lift the towel over your head.*

5 *Rotate your arms further behind your head for another, even deeper, set. Bring your arms to the front again.*

6 *Lift your arms overhead, bend your knees, and lower your arms down.*

Do's and don'ts
* Keep your shoulders even. Don't allow one shoulder to lift or hunch forward. * Don't release your ribcage to the front or let your back sway.
* Keep your spine elongated and your abdominal muscles actively contracted to support your torso.

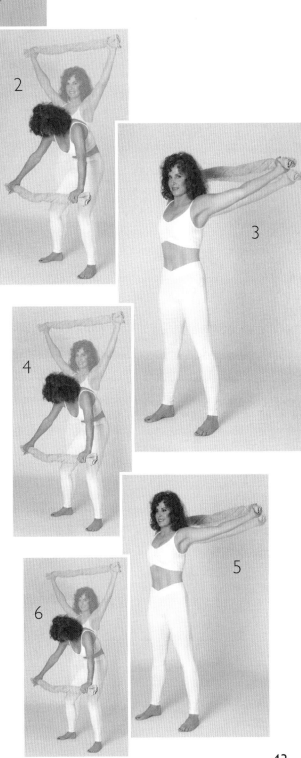

43

Backward stretch and lift

The object of this exercise is to build a stable shoulder system for everyday actions, such as lifting, pushing, or rotating, that can develop muscle imbalances. In order to equalize your muscles, you need to practice movements that protect your joints while uniformly strengthening the muscles in your chest, upper back, and arms.

Breathing pattern

• Inhale twice as you bend your arms. Exhale twice as you bring them down behind you.

• Inhale twice as you raise your arms above you. Exhale at the top.

Do's and don'ts
* Use your upper back and chest muscles to prevent your shoulders from lifting at the same time as your arms. * Anchor your pelvis to avoid arching your lower back as you bring your arms behind your back. * Keep movements fluid, but your body still.

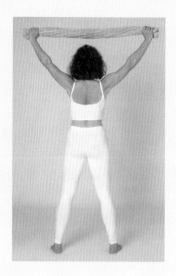

Starting position
Stand with your feet apart. Bring the towel over your head, pulling it taut. Relax your shoulders and engage your back muscles to keep tension out of your neck.

Variation
Keep your towel loose, not taut. To begin your movement, you can release the stretch of your towel as you lower it behind your back and as you lift it up, stretching it out only at the bottom and top of the exercise. To increase the stretch, bring the towel behind your back and stretch it away from your torso as you lower it.

Repetitions
Repeat the exercise eight times.

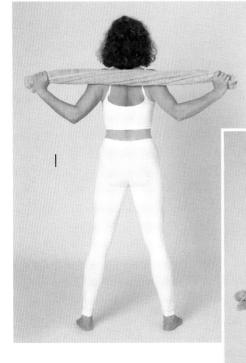

What you should feel
As tension is relieved, your upper body
strength will be balanced by your flexibility.

1 *Bend your arms, pulling your
elbows toward your waist and
keeping the towel taut.*

2 *Straighten your arms behind
your back, bringing the towel
down to your waist.*

3 *Bend your elbows as you
bring the towel up to your
head. Keep it taut and then
straighten your arms to lift
it above your head.*

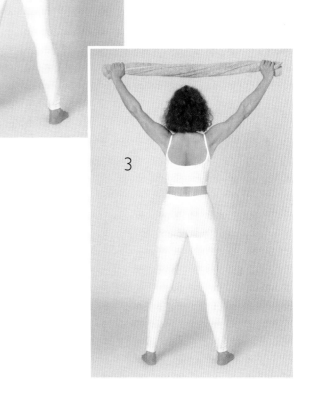

45

Small presses up

This exercise continues to work through your full range of motion in order to bring about total chest opening and upper torso flexibility. It loosens the tight chest muscles that affect posture and strengthens the upper back.

Breathing pattern

• Take a full breath as you lift the towel over your head and bring it behind your back.

• Use a double inhale and double exhale breathing pattern for the pulses.

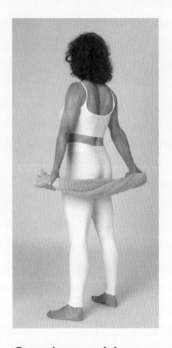

What you should feel
The blood circulation to the upper chest and shoulders will create heat in the muscles.

Starting position
Stand with your feet apart. With your arms straight, hold the towel behind your buttocks.

Variation
Never release your ribcage forward to increase the range of motion to your back. This can compress the lower back muscles and spine. Range of motion will only increase when the torso alignment is stable and anchored. Work for full mobility with core stabilization for maximum benefits.

Repetitions
Repeat the exercise three times.

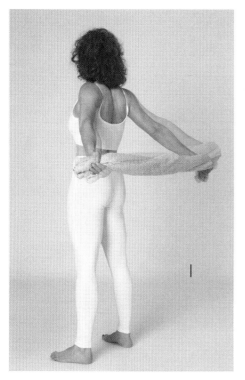

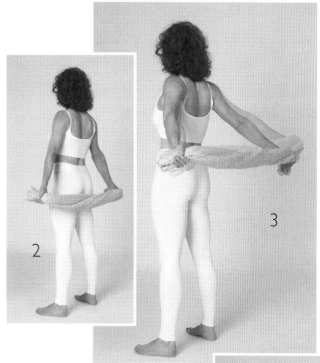

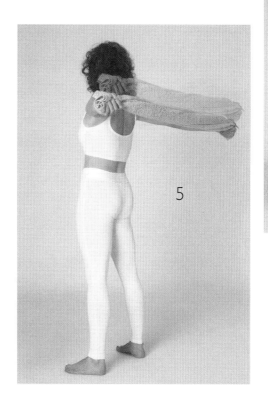

1 Keep your arms straight and lift them up behind your back to hip level. Without leaning forward, pulse your arms upward with eight small pulses.

2 Lower the towel behind your buttocks again.

3 Lift your arms to waist level and pulse upward eight times.

4 Lower the towel behind your buttocks again.

5 Lift your arms as high as you comfortably can behind your back, maintaining your alignment in your torso. Pulse upward eight times and then lower your arms again.

Arm, back, and chest stretch

The purpose of this exercise is to strengthen the muscles around the shoulders without straining the joints themselves. Active stretching prepares your body for movement and helps to prevent muscle and joint injury. Keeping your shoulder joints lubricated and the muscles and tendons around the joints mobile helps to eliminate stress and strain.

Breathing pattern

• Inhale twice as you bring the towel down behind your back.

• Exhale twice as you lift the towel over your head.

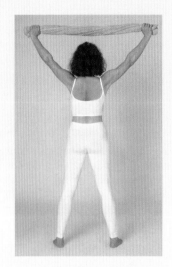

Starting position
Stand with your feet apart. Raise your arms over your head, pulling the towel taut. Press your shoulders down and away from your ears. Keep your head in line with your spine.

What you should feel
Both your posture and circulation will improve, and you should feel tightness in your upper body disappearing and its range of motion increasing.

Do's and don'ts
* Don't lift your shoulders as the towel comes up and back; if you need to, grab the towel at the ends. * Don't lift or press your ribcage forward. * Keep your torso and buttocks in support of the alignment. * Keep your chin up and smile.

Repetitions
Repeat the exercise eight times.

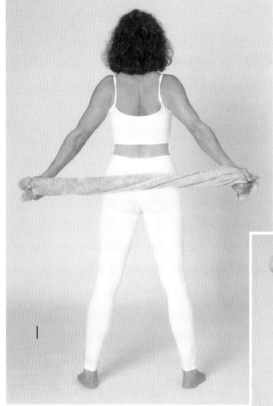

1 *With your arms straight, bring the taut towel down behind your back.*

2 *With your arms straight, raise the taut towel upward and over your head.*

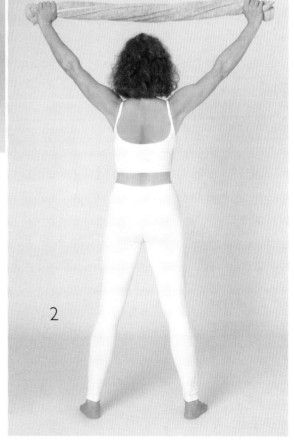

Side stretch

Most everyday activities are one-sided, creating imbalances that misalign our bodies. This side stretch can help to balance the strength of the muscles on both sides of your body, as well as helping you to become more flexible.

Breathing pattern

- Exhale twice as you stretch to the side.

- Inhale twice as you lift to the center.

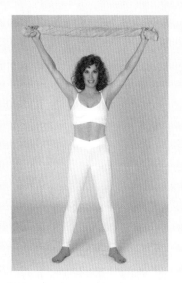

Starting position

Stand with your feet apart. Raise your arms over your head, pulling the towel taut and keeping it centered above your head. If, when you look up, you can see the towel, you are rounding your shoulders and losing your core alignment.

What you should feel
Your torso muscles will stretch and lengthen, and your core muscles will become balanced.

Do's and don'ts
* Keep your hips aligned and support the bend by tightening the muscles of your buttocks and stomach. * Lift up and off your hips as you bend over, as if you are reaching for the ceiling. * Don't twist your shoulders, but keep them in a straight line, with your chest open and your shoulder blades back and down.

Repetitions
Repeat the stretch four times, alternating sides.

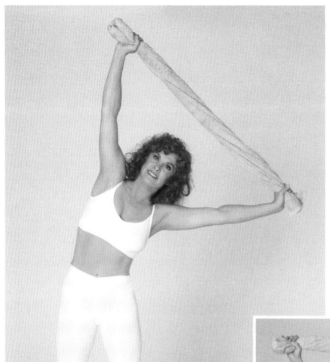

Variation
Divide your stretch into four parts and stretch slowly over to the side. Inhale and exhale as you stretch. Stay in the side-stretch position and take a full breath, contracting deeply on the bending side and elongating the stretching side. This will intensify your waistline work.

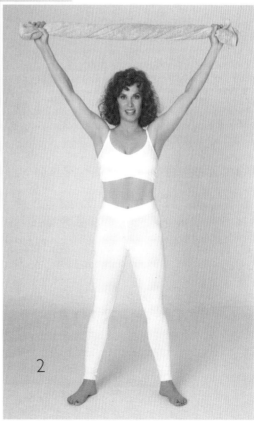

1 *Lift up your torso by increasing the distance between your hips and ribcage. Stretch your body over to one side, keeping your shoulders and hips in a straight line.*

2 *Lift up your torso and return to the standing position. Repeat the stretch on the other side.*

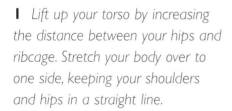

Side stretch with cross arm

Retraining your muscles to form new healthy movement patterns takes focus, attentiveness, and time. When you properly repeat a movement pattern, your muscles remember, reinforcing the mind–body connection. Concentrating on the alignment of this exercise will determine how quickly your muscles respond to new patterns.

This exercise is a deeper side stretch which requires more concentration to maintain the alignment. The deeper you go in the stretch, the deeper you will be able to go.

Breathing pattern

• Inhale twice and exhale twice as you stretch to the side.

• Inhale twice and exhale twice as you reach across your body.

• Inhale twice and exhale twice as you touch the towel.

• Inhale twice and exhale twice as you lift your torso up to the center.

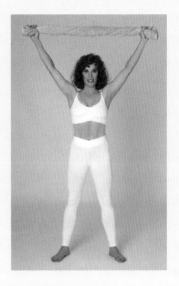

Starting position
Stand with your feet apart. Raise your arms over your head, pulling the towel taut.

Do's and don'ts
* Stabilize your shoulders and your hips. * Don't rotate your shoulders and hips, as this will cause discomfort in your back or knees. * Stretch only as far as you can while maintaining your core postural alignment. * Always reach up and out as you bend over and keep the overhead arm reaching toward the side wall.

1 Stretch your upper body over to one side, keeping your hips and shoulders in a straight line. Count slowly to four as you stretch over.

2 Release your lower hand from the towel and reach your arm across your body. Keep your shoulders in alignment and your head in line with your spine.

3 Sweep your arm to touch the towel. Repeat the arm movement four times.

4 Hold the towel taut with both hands and raise your torso to the standing position.

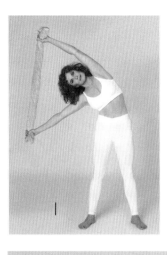

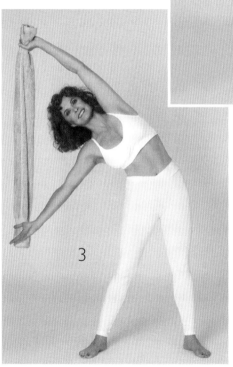

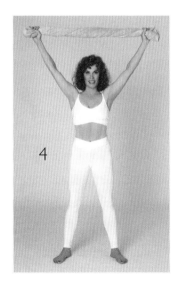

What you should feel
As you are able to go deeper into the stretch you will feel your muscles release in the waist and hips while you are maintaining support. You should also feel your torso muscles lengthen.

Overhead twist

Rotating your torso will improve the flexibility of your spine and give you the strength and mobility you need for any activity. This exercise has the added benefit of keeping your body youthful, whatever your age.

Breathing pattern

• Using the double inhale and double exhale pattern, take four breaths with the four counts as you twist to the side and twist to the center.

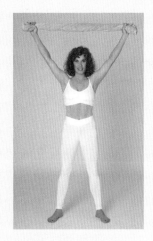

Starting position

Stand with your feet apart. Lift the towel over your head. Keep your body weight evenly distributed on both your feet, maintaining your foot triangles (see p.14).

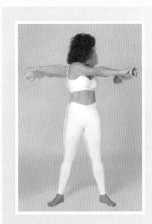

Variation

If holding the towel over your head is too difficult, hold it in front of your chest instead.

To advance the level of the exercise, add eight small yet quick pulses from your waist after twisting to the side.

Repetitions

Repeat the exercise four times, alternating sides.

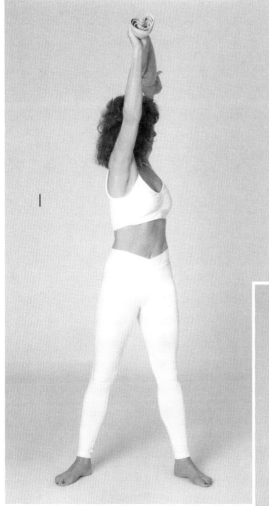

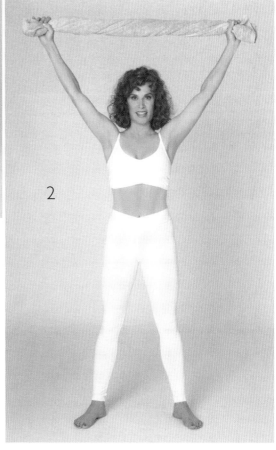

1 *Anchor your hips to the front and, counting to four, twist at your waist to the left side. Remember to keep the towel over the center of your head.*

2 *Twist to the center, counting to four as you return to the starting position. Repeat the sequence to the right side.*

55

Hip pulses

Stretching the hip joints and working the muscles attached to them is crucial to the way you stand, walk, and sit. This exercise reveals imbalances in the way you move your hips in daily life. Most people find that one hip is extremely mobile while the other barely moves. Work your tighter hip first and you will find that this movement helps you to begin to balance your body when you stand.

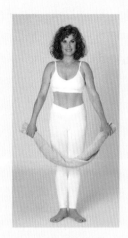

Starting position
Stand with your heels together and your toes apart. Hold the towel in front of you.

Breathing pattern

• Inhale twice as you stretch to the side and exhale twice as you press through the center.

• Inhale and exhale twice as you pulse your hips.

What you should feel
You should feel your hip joints releasing and giving you better support while you are standing.

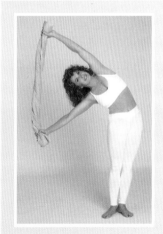

Variation
Once you have achieved the evenness of movement in your hips, lift your arm over your head and stretch away from the towel. Open your chest and twist toward the ceiling, looking up and behind your towel. Repeat this movement four times before returning to the center position and doing the movement on the opposite side.

Do's and don'ts
* Bend directly over the side. * Don't twist your hips * Keep the muscles of your buttocks and stomach tightly contracted for support.

Repetitions
Repeat the exercise twice.

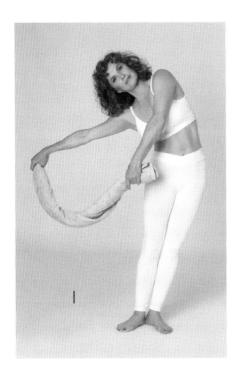

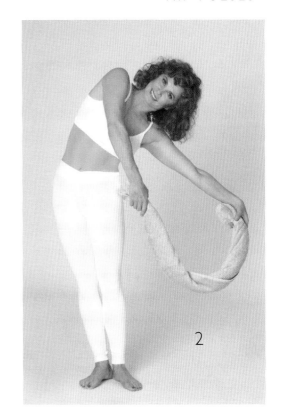

1 *Press your hip to one side, lengthening the space from the hip to your shoulder and contracting the opposite side of your body. Keep your head in line with your spine and stretch your arms away from your torso at the side of your body.*

2 *Press through the center and repeat the exercise on the other side.*

Repeat Steps 1 and 2, and add eight quick, small pulses from the hip bones.

3 *Repeat the exercise again, pressing further over to each side and lifting your arms to shoulder level. Add the eight hip pulses, pressing through the center.*

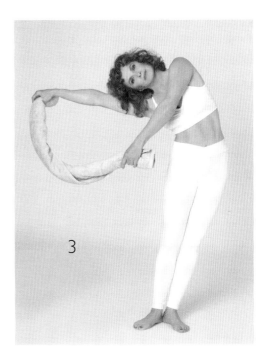

4 Mat and floorwork

* The hundred

* Diamond to roll-up

* Roll-up to diamond

* Diamond spine roll

* Traditional roll-up

* Hip lifts with leg circles

* Single leg pull

* Single-leg side stretch

* Double leg pull

* Double-leg side stretch

* Straight leg pull

* Leg stretch and arm reach

Now it's time to get down to working on the floor. You will need to lie or sit on the floor for all these exercises, so soften your working surface with a yoga mat or another soft but firm mat that is not likely to slide or bunch up. Whatever mat you choose, make sure that it is the right size and that its thickness is comfortable for you.

We start with a classic sequence called "the hundred", which builds center body strength. The next series of Pilates exercises includes roll-ups, spine rolls, hip lifts, leg pulls, side stretches, and leg stretches that increase the flexibility of your spine, tone the muscles in your abdomen and legs, and build core stability and strength.

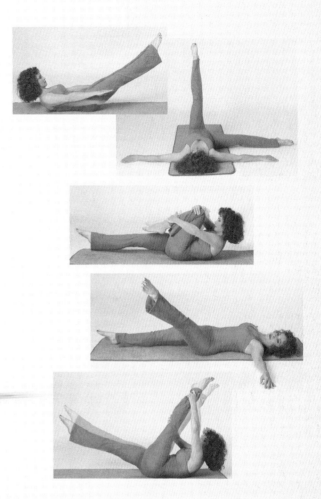

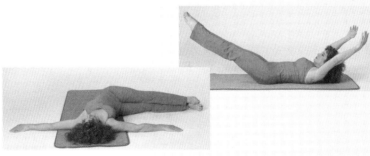

The hundred

This classic Pilates exercise is so named because it takes a count of 100 to complete. It stimulates the circulation, strengthens core alignment, stabilizes the trunk muscles, and expands the chest and ribcage. During the exercise, your abdominal muscles must stay scooped and your back must remain flat on the floor as you lower your legs.

The most important aspect of this exercise is to keep your lower back pressed firmly into the mat and your abdominal muscles pulled inward to support your back. You may need to keep your knees bent in order to maintain your spinal alignment.

Decrease the number of repetitions if you feel any tension in your neck or discomfort in your lower back. As you progress, make sure the transition to the next position is intentional and never allows your back to lift from the mat.

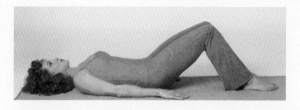

Starting position
Lie with knees bent, bringing toes, ankles, and knees together.

Breathing pattern

• Inhale and exhale to lift your upper body off the mat and pulse downward. Use small breaths for each beat of the arms, with five inhales and five exhales. If this is too difficult at first, use a pattern of two inhales and two exhales. Add more breath as you progress with the exercise.

• Inhale and exhale to lower your upper body and place your feet on the mat.

What you should feel
Your breathing will improve, your trunk muscles will stabilize, and your abdominal muscles will feel toned.

Repetitions
Complete only one sequence of this exercise.

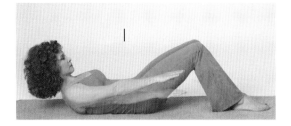

1 Lift your upper body, shoulders, neck, and head off the mat by tightening your abdominal muscles and stabilizing your back and pelvis. Pull your navel toward your spine. Reach toward your toes, pulling your shoulders away from your ears and pressing your shoulder blades into the mat. Using a small pumping movement, pulse your arms up and down about 15cm (6in).

Match your breathing to your pumping movements, inhaling five times and exhaling five times. Stay in this position for a count of 20.

2 Slowly lift your legs off the floor to a 90° angle. Continue the pumping movements and the breathing pattern for a count of 20.

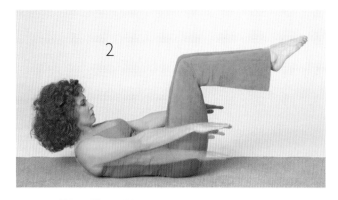

3 Slowly extend your legs toward the ceiling and keep pumping for a further count of 20.

4 Begin to lower your legs at a diagonal to your torso and carry out a further count of 20.

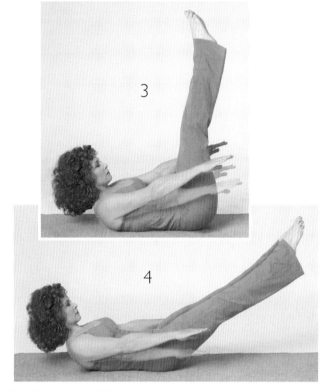

5 Finally, lower your legs as close to the ground as possible without allowing your spine to lift off the mat, and complete the hundred with your last count of 20. This is optional and more advanced.

Lower your head to the mat. Release your arms, bend your knees, and place your feet on the mat.

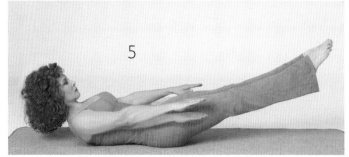

Diamond to roll-up

This exercise works the muscles of your abdomen and lubricates your spine. The aim is to place your spine on the mat, one vertebra at a time, with full abdominal control. This can take years to master, but it improves postural alignment and keeps your abdominal muscles functionally strong. You will also learn to focus and concentrate deeply inside your body in order to maintain balance.

Breathing pattern

• Inhale as you bring your legs into the diamond. Exhale as you stretch forward.

• Inhale for a count of four as you roll back, straightening your legs.

• Exhale for a count of four as you circle your arms around and roll up, bringing your legs back to the diamond position.

• Exhale for a count of four as you stretch forward.

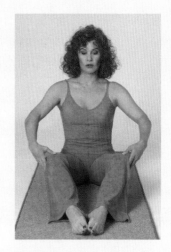

Starting position
Bring your feet together and bend your knees to form a diamond shape with your legs. Sit tall and lengthen your spine upward. Place your hands lightly on your knees.

What you should feel
Your back muscles will be more flexible and your abdomen should feel toned.

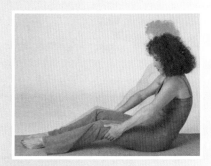

Variation
At first, you may need to place both your hands under your thighs to help you support your torso as you roll back and up.

Repetitions
Repeat the exercise three times.

1 *Contract your abdominal muscles and round your back, stretching your torso toward your feet. Pull your navel toward your spine as you work your body in opposition.*

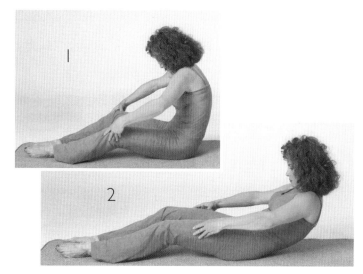

2 *Slowly move back, rolling one vertebra at a time. As you roll back, straighten your legs, bring your knees together and stretch your torso away from your legs.*

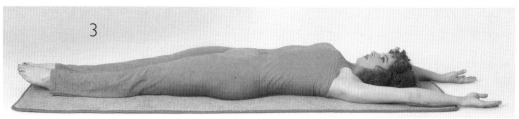

3 *Lower your head to the mat. Reach your arms over your head, placing them on the floor.*

4 *Circle both your arms around the sides of your body to the front and lift your head, neck, and shoulders. Close your ribs and tighten your abdominal muscles.*

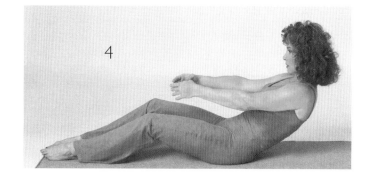

5 *Roll your torso up from the mat, rolling one vertebra at a time and returning to the diamond position.*

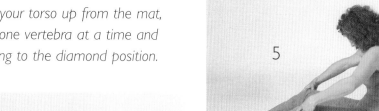

Don't
* lift your shoulders
* lose support in the abdomen or you will injure your back

Roll-up to diamond

This exercise helps you to build up abdominal strength and improve the flexibility of your spine. Strong abdominal muscles and a supple back keep your body vital, youthful, and healthy.

Breathing pattern

• Inhale for a count of four as you roll up and exhale for a count of four as you roll down.

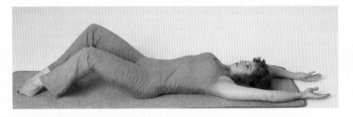

Starting position

Lie with your legs in the diamond position and your arms on the floor above your head. Keep each vertebra on the mat to "imprint" your spine.

I *Lift your arms toward the ceiling, engaging the upper back muscles and closing the ribcage. Lift your head, neck, and shoulders, and begin to move upward, slowly peeling your spine from the mat and looking down.*

2 *Extend your legs as you roll upward.*

3 *Stretch your torso over your legs, keeping your abdominal muscles pulled upward and your navel pulled in toward your spine. Create a C shape with your body. Hold your arms directly around your ears.*

4 *Begin to roll back down on to the mat, pulling your legs into the diamond position as you move.*

5 *Lift your arms above your head and finally place your head on the floor, with your body in the starting position.*

Repetitions
Repeat the exercise three times.

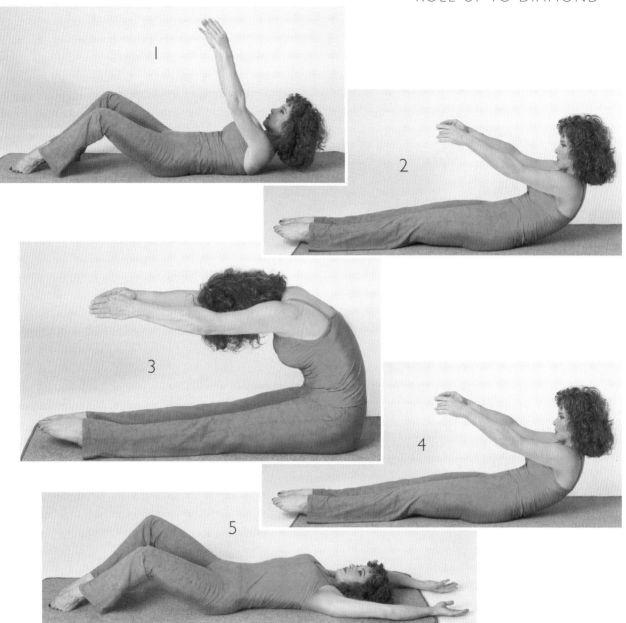

Do's and don'ts
* Keep the movement fluid and constant. * Pull your abdominal muscles inward and upward, away from your legs. * Hollow your low abdominal muscles as you roll. * Don't straighten your spine. * If you feel any stress in your back or neck, hold on to your thighs until you are stronger.

65

Diamond spine roll

In the last two exercises, your legs moved with the roll of the torso. In this exercise, you keep the diamond position throughout for more powerful work in your core muscles. Balance the concave shape of the abdomen with the convex shape of the spine. Keep the roundness of the torso while rolling down and rolling up.

Breathing pattern

• Exhale for a count of four as you contract and roll to the floor.

• Inhale for a count of four as you circle your arms around and roll up.

• Exhale for a count of four as you roll up.

Do's and don'ts
* Keep your stomach contracted for support.
* Don't lose contact with the floor.

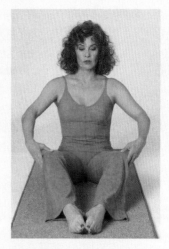

Starting position
Bring your feet together and bend your knees to form a diamond with your legs. Lengthen your spine and stretch the space between the top of your hips and the bottom of your ribcage.

Variation
If you have difficulty rolling up, begin by sitting tall and placing your hands under your thighs. Contract your abdominal muscles and round your back, keeping your shoulders directly over your hips. Pull the muscles inward and upward to form the C shape. Straighten your back. Exhale as you contract and inhale as you lengthen your spine.

Repetitions
Repeat the exercise three times.

1 Contract your abdominal muscles and round your back, stretching your torso toward your feet. Pull your navel to your spine and pull your lower abdominal muscles inward and upward.

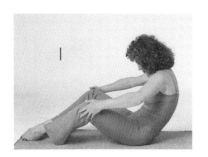

2 Begin to roll your back down, keeping it rounded and close to the floor. As you roll back, stretch your torso away from your legs.

3 Lower your head to the mat and reach your arms above your head to the floor.

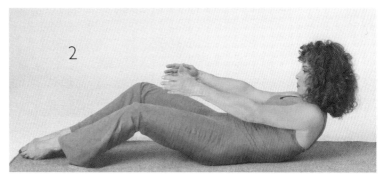

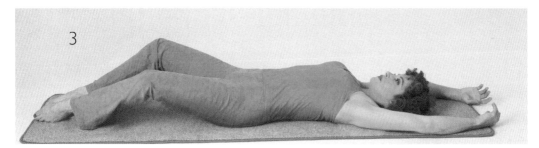

4 Circle your arms around to the sides of your body to the front and lift your head, neck, and shoulders. Roll your torso up from the mat, articulating your spine by rolling one vertebra at a time. Keep your back rounded as you stretch over your legs

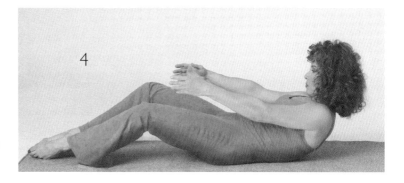

What you should feel
Your abdominal muscles will become flatter and feel toned.

Traditional roll-up

The traditional roll-up combines core stabilization with spinal flexion and muscle control to align the spine and strengthen the abdominal muscles. With each repetition, try to keep your lower body still and anchored to the floor. The more fully you inhale and exhale, the deeper you engage your abdominal muscles. Because your head is a heavy weight, look and reach for your toes as you lift it in order to prevent strain.

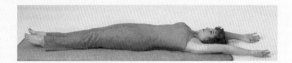

Starting position
Lie with your legs straight and arms on the floor above your head. Imprint your spine, keeping each vertebra on the mat.

Breathing pattern

• Inhale for a count of two as you lift your arms to the ceiling.

• Exhale for a count of four as you pull your abdomen inward and begin to roll up and over your legs.

• Inhale as you flex your feet.

• Exhale for a count of four as you begin to roll back down.

• Inhale and exhale in position.

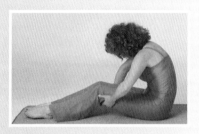

Variation
Start the exercise with your knees bent, supported by your hands, and your feet flat on the floor. Sit very tall and stretch your arms out in front of you. Inhale and lengthen your spine. Strongly exhale as you contract your abdominal muscles and roll back toward the mat. Keep the movement controlled and roll only as far as you can with your abdomen scooped. Inhale as you return to the sitting position.

What you should feel
You should feel your back muscles stretching, more flexibility in your spine, and increased abdominal strength.

Repetitions
Repeat the exercise five times.

1 *Lift your arms toward the ceiling, engaging your upper back muscles and closing your ribcage. Curl your head, neck, and shoulders off the mat and continue to roll up slowly. Scoop your abdomen back toward your spine and roll up like a wheel, curling your torso off the mat.*

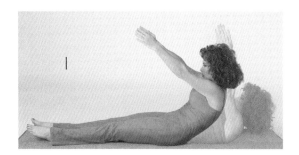

2 *Bring your torso over your legs and stretch your fingertips toward your toes or the wall, with your arms around your ears. Stretch forward from the hips and keep your shoulders down, away from your ears. Flex your feet and anchor them to the mat.*

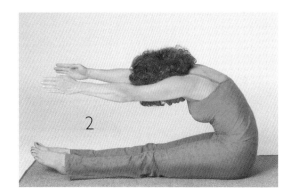

3 *Begin to roll back down, pulling away from your legs. Imprint your spine on to the mat, one vertebra at a time. Stretch your spine, shoulders, neck, and head to the floor.*

4 *Stretch your arms above your head to the floor and relax.*

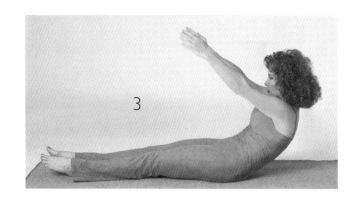

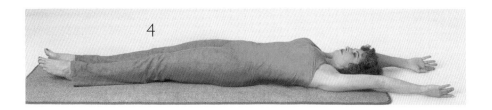

Hip lifts with leg circles

This exercise simulates the motion of the hip joints when we walk. Performing the motion while lying down changes the gravitational force on the joints and muscles involved in walking. This helps to balance asymmetrical movements and evenly lubricate the joints.

Breathing pattern

- Inhale twice as you lift up your hip.

- Exhale twice as you lower your hip to the mat.

- Inhale twice as you extend your bent leg to the ceiling.

- As you circle in one direction, inhale for a count of five, then exhale for a count of five as you circle in the other direction.

- For the large circles, inhale and exhale for a count of five.

Variation
If you cannot straighten your leg to the ceiling, work with your knee bent at a 90° angle and keep your circles small and precise.

Repetitions
Complete the sequence once, then repeat with the other leg.

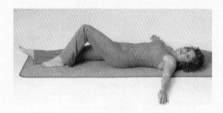

Starting position
Lie with your spine imprinted on the mat and your legs straight. Place your arms on the floor away from your body, with your palms down. Bend one leg.

Do's and don'ts
* Keep your shoulders and lower back pressed to the mat for support. * Don't over-extend the leg so that you lift your lower back off the mat.

What you should feel
Your hips joints should feel more flexible and your inner and outer thigh muscles toned.

1 *Press the foot of your bent leg into the floor as you lift the hip up and toward the center. Don't let your knee move with the hip. Press the hip down on to the mat. Repeat five times.*

2 *Extend the leg toward the ceiling at a 90° angle to your pelvis, pressing your lower back into the mat.*

3 *Keep your hips completely still and make a small circle with your leg across your body. The smaller the circle, the deeper the movement will be in the hip joint. Circle five times. Then circle in the opposite direction five times. The hip is now prepared for the large leg circles.*

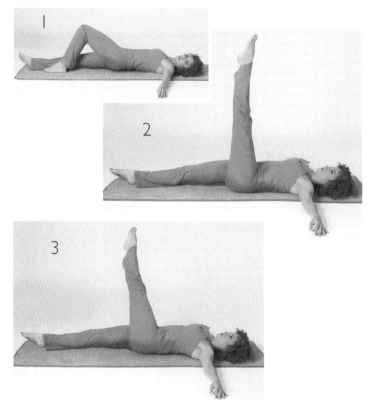

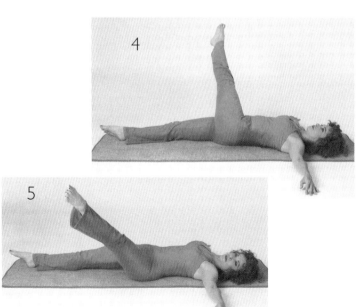

4 *Extend the leg across your body as far as possible without losing the control and stillness in the opposing hip and leg.*

5 *Sweep the leg down to the opposing leg and then back across in a large circle, extending the leg out at the side of your body. Anchor your torso at your hips and keep them level.*

Repeat the leg circles five times, then repeat them five times in the opposite direction.

Single leg pull

The single leg pull coordinates mind, body, and breath with an exercise for the whole body. It balances both sides of the body, flexes and extends the spine, and matches breath to movement at the same time.

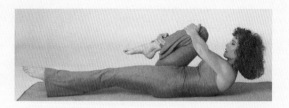

Breathing pattern

• Inhale twice as you bring your knee in toward your chest.

• Exhale twice as you extend and swap legs.

Starting position

Lie with your spine imprinted on the mat and your legs straight. Bend one knee and bring the leg toward your chest. Lift your upper back and head, and place your outside hand on your ankle. Place the other hand on your knee. Lift the extended leg off the mat to hip level. Keep your spine imprinted on the mat.

What you should feel

Your legs and abdominal muscles will feel toned and your leg and back muscles stretched.

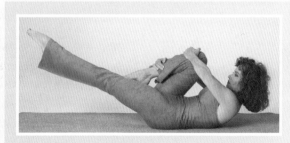

Variation

If you cannot keep your spine flat on your mat, lift your extended leg toward the ceiling. The nearer your legs are to the floor, the more difficult the exercise becomes.

Repetitions

Repeat the whole exercise eight times.

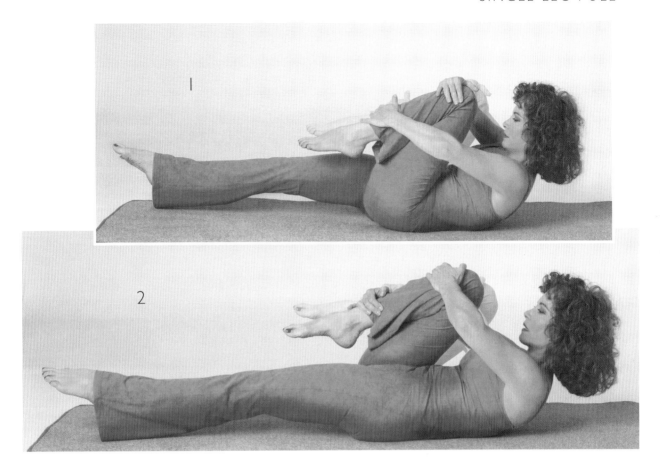

1 *Pulse the bent knee toward your shoulder twice, while contracting your upper abdominal muscles and reaching your shoulders toward your knee.*

2 *Extend the leg until it is straight and repeat the exercise with your other leg.*

Do's and don'ts
* Stretch the extended leg past the other leg, reaching a little farther each time. * Don't kick your legs away from your body, but fully extend them from your core. * Keep your abdominal muscles pressed to your spine. * Keep your spine imprinted on the mat. * Don't lift your chin. * Focus your eyes on your knees, stretching the back of your neck. * Keep the extended leg reaching for the wall.

Single-leg side stretch

This stretching exercise rotates the ball-and-socket joint of each hip in order to maximize its range of motion. This is not a simple leg lift, but a movement that comes from deep within your core abdominal strength. This is especially true as you lift your leg toward the ceiling.

Breathing pattern

• Take one full breath to lower your leg and one full breath to lift your leg toward the ceiling.

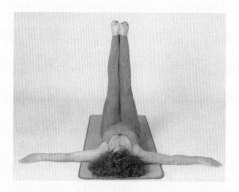

Starting position

Lie with your spine imprinted on the mat and your legs straight. Extend your arms and rest them on the floor with your palms down. Bend your knees to your chest and extend them to the ceiling at a 90° angle, directly above your hips. Engage your shoulder blades to actively press your upper back and shoulders to the mat. For stability, do not lose support from your abdomen.

What you should feel

You should feel a tremendous stretching of the inner thigh and a release of the ball-and-socket joint of each hip. You will also feel a great deal of circulation in the abdomen if you have properly maintained support by tightening the muscles. Your back between the shoulder blades will feel lighter as a result of your stabilization work.

Variation

Tight hamstring muscles or tightness in your hips and back may prevent you from straightening your legs or stretching all the way to the floor. Bend your knees to a 90° angle and perform the exercise with your knees bent until you can work with them in the straight position.

Repetitions

Repeat the whole exercise four times.

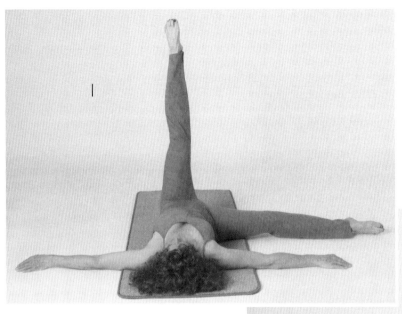

1 Lower one leg to the floor at the side of your body and at hip level. Allow your other hip to lift only enough to let the lowering foot touch the floor. Keep your lifted leg stretched toward the ceiling.

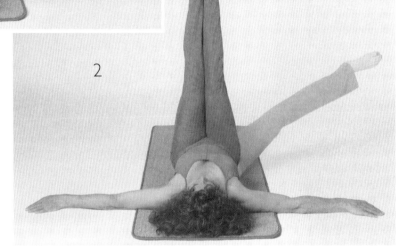

2 Tighten your abdominal muscles and roll the small of your back to the floor while lifting and returning your leg toward the ceiling.

3 Press both hips evenly to the floor before beginning the exercise on the other side.

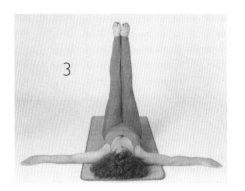

Double leg pull

This exercise aims to develop core stability in your spine. It involves extending your arms and legs away from your center, and uses your abdominal muscles to achieve both strength and endurance.

Breathing pattern

• Inhale twice as you press your legs toward your chest.

• Fully exhale as you extend your legs and arms. Continue to exhale as you circle your arms and bend your knees. This long exhale is meant to squeeze all the air out of your lungs so that you can fully inhale to replenish and energize your system.

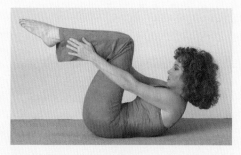

Starting position

Lie with your spine imprinted on the mat and your legs straight. Bend your knees toward your chest. Contract your abdominal muscles, lift your upper back and head, and place your hands on your legs above your ankles. Anchor your core alignment to the mat.

Variation
If your back begins to lift from the mat, or your abdominal muscles jut out, extend your legs higher toward the ceiling. If your neck muscles tire, use more upper abdominal control and do not stretch your arms back, but lift them toward the ceiling.

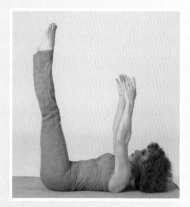

What you should feel
Your spine should feel stronger and your leg and abdominal muscles toned.

Repetitions
Repeat the exercise four times.

1 *Move your legs toward your chest with two small presses.*

2 *Extend your legs on a diagonal line. At the same time, straighten your arms and stretch them past your ears.*

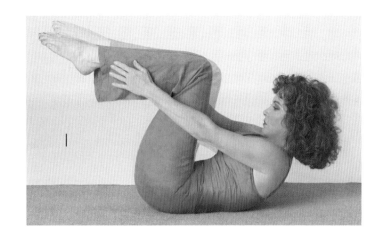

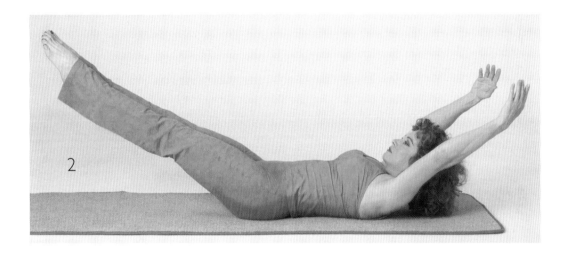

3 *Circle your extended arms around to your sides, while bending your knees toward your chest.*

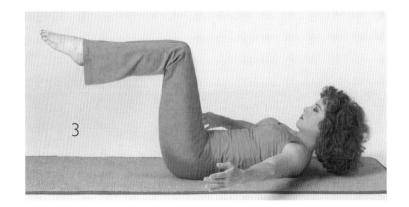

Double-leg side stretch

This exercise further develops your practice of side rotation and hip opening. Use your core muscles to perform these precise and powerful movements in order for the work to penetrate deeply into the hip joints.

Breathing pattern

- Inhale and exhale after you lift your legs to the starting position.

- Exhale twice as you lower your right leg.

- Inhale twice as you lower your left leg.

- Exhale twice as you lift your left leg.

- Inhale twice as you lift your right leg.

- Exhale and inhale and repeat.

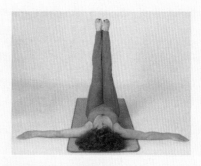

Starting position

Lie with your spine imprinted on the mat and your legs straight. Extend your arms out and place them on the floor, with the palms down. Bend your knees to your chest and extend them toward the ceiling at a 90° angle, directly above your hips. Relax and lengthen your neck muscles.

Do's and don'ts

* Don't let your shoulders lose contact with the mat.
* Press your shoulders and upper back to the mat for support.

What you should feel

Your hips will feel more flexible, your torso stretched, and your legs toned.

Variation

Perform the exercise with your knees bent to a 90° angle until you can work with your legs in the straight position.

Repetitions

Repeat the whole exercise four times.

I *Lower one leg to the floor at the side of your body at hip level. Keep the other leg lifted, allowing the hip to lift from the floor.*

2 *Bring the raised leg down on top of the first leg. Press your shoulders firmly to the floor and feel the stretch in opposition across your body.*

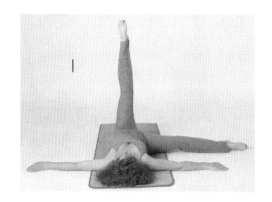

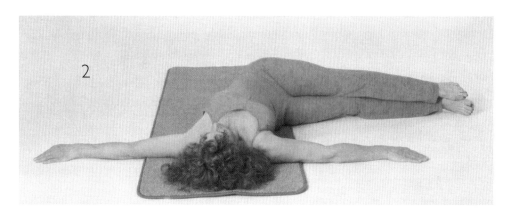

3 *Lift the top leg toward the ceiling again by rolling the hip, not by swinging the leg.*

4 *Tighten your abdominal muscles, roll the small of your back to the floor, and lift the remaining leg toward the ceiling. Press both hips evenly to the floor before beginning the exercise on the other side.*

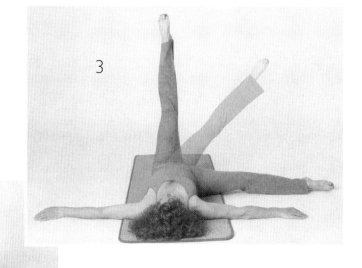

Straight leg pull

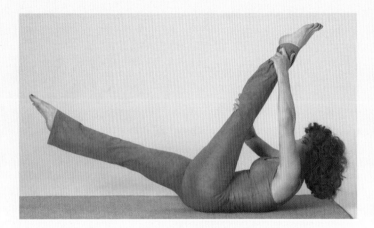

You must be careful to concentrate on maintaining balance through the core strength you have been using. Feel the breathing deeply and engage your abdominal muscles to lift your upper torso toward your leg. This is an intense posture and the benefits are very profound. You will have to pay attention to the position of your head in order not to strain your neck.

Breathing pattern

- Double inhale as you pulse your leg.

- Exhale once as you swap legs.

Starting position

Lie with your spine imprinted on the mat and your legs straight. Bend your knees and bring them toward your chest. Extend your legs toward the ceiling at a 90° angle, directly up from your hips. Lift your upper back and head. Lower one leg until it hovers at eye level and hold the ankle and calf of the raised leg. Scoop your abdominal muscles to flatten your abdomen.

Repetitions
Repeat the exercise eight times, alternating sides.

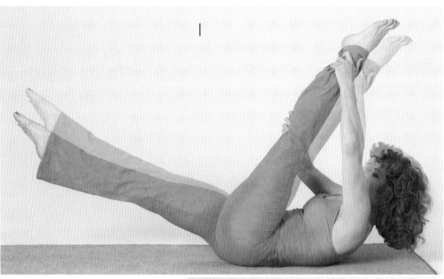

1 *Lift your upper torso toward your raised leg as you pulse the leg twice.*

2 *Switch legs and repeat the exercise.*

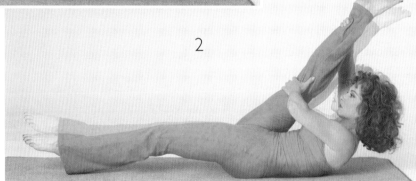

What you should feel
The body control you will feel is directly related to the strength you have and it will build as you become stronger. There is a wonderful feeling of accomplishment when you can execute this posture correctly.

Variation
With your spine imprinted and your shoulders and hips anchored, lower the leg only as far as you can. A smaller range of motion and fewer repetitions may be necessary until you build up core strength.

Leg stretch and arm reach

This movement increases the flexibility of your spine and improves the circulation in the upper back muscles that support your spinal column. Turning your head is very important as it strengthens your neck muscles and alleviates tension in your neck. Make each breath match a movement, using more breaths to slow a movement down rather than rush through it.

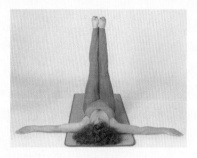

Starting position

Lie with your spine imprinted on the mat and your legs straight. Place your arms on the floor at your sides, palms down. Bend your knees to your chest and extend them toward the ceiling at a 90° angle, directly above your hips. Relax and lengthen your neck muscles.

Breathing pattern

- Exhale as you lower your leg to the floor.

- Inhale as you lower your other leg.

- Exhale as you bring one arm over to the other.

- Inhale as you lift your arm back toward the ceiling and place it on the floor.

- Exhale as you lift your leg toward the ceiling.

- Inhale as you lift your other leg and return it to the starting position.

What you should feel
Your hips and torso should feel more flexible, with your legs toned, and your arms and back muscles stretched.

Variation
To make this exercise more advanced, perform it slowly, taking two or three breaths to stretch to each position. Each time you reach to the side, try to stretch a little further than the last, keeping arms and legs straight.

Repetitions
Repeat the exercise four times, alternating sides.

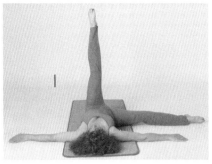

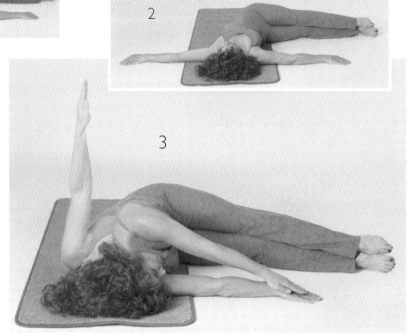

1 *Lower a leg to the floor at hip level. Let the hip of the raised leg lift from the floor.*

2 *Lower the raised leg down on top of your other leg and keep both straight at hip level.*

3 *Lift the outside arm, raise the shoulder, and roll toward your legs, reaching out your arms and hands. Turn your gaze slowly to follow the movement of your hands.*

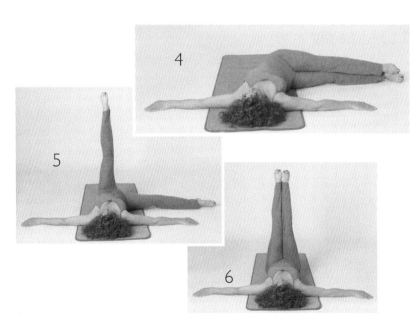

4 *Lift up the same arm and roll across your back. Place your shoulder, arm, and hand on the floor, bringing your head into the center position.*

5 *Bring your top leg back toward the ceiling.*

6 *Tighten your abdominal muscles, roll the small of your back on the floor, and bring the remaining leg to join the first. Press both hips evenly to the floor.*

5 Advanced mat and floorwork

* Rolling like a ball

* Leg extensions

* Open-leg rocker

* Flex and point release

* Spine stretch

* Twist

* Twist with arm presses

* Saw

* Saw with arm presses

* Circle in the sand

* Flat presses

* Knee twist

* Side stretch

* Single push-up

* Side leg-kick series
  – *point up, flex down*
  – *pulse to sweep*
  – *bicycle*
  – *beats with point and flex*

* Roll-up to alignment

* Cool down

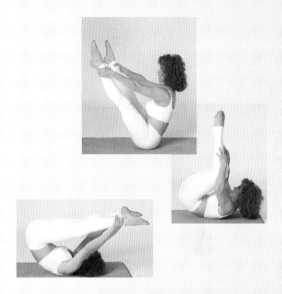

Your floorwork moves into a more advanced stage with the emphasis on whole-body movement. Initially, you need to focus on the "ball" position, which you use for rolling through the movement.

After some leg extensions and small abdominal contractions, you move on to the open-leg rocker, which will tell you which side of your body is dominant or if you have any imbalances. There follows a sequence of spine stretches, twists, saws, and push-ups before you engage in the side leg-kick series. This is composed of four movements that are brilliantly designed to stretch, tone, strengthen, and lengthen the leg muscles simultaneously. They create the long, lean muscles of a dancer's legs and focus on pelvic stabilization, which is essential for healthy backs, hips, and knees.

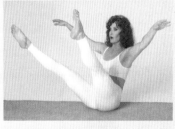

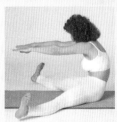

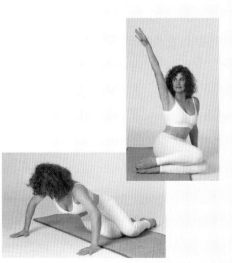

Rolling like a ball

This classic example of a Pilates whole-body movement mobilizes and restores the natural alignment of the spine. Controlling your shape and ensuring your vertebrae move smoothly, or articulate, together are key to its success. This will enable you to use your core abdominal strength, rather than momentum, to roll through the movement. If you feel any flat spots in your back, roll more slowly and try to stretch each vertebra as you move.

Breathing pattern

• Inhale as you roll back.

• Exhale as you roll up.

What you should feel
You should feel a tremendous release in the back and a stretching of the spine. You will also feel a strengthening of the lower abdomen.

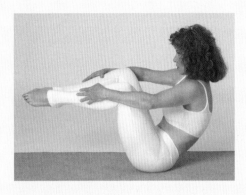

Starting position
Sit down and bend your knees to your chest. Rest your hands on your lower legs. Lift your legs off the mat and open your knees until they are shoulder-distance apart. Keep your feet together. Deeply contract the muscles in your abdomen and curve your back. Bring your head toward your knees so that it follows the roundness of your spine.

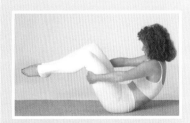

Variation
If you cannot perform the rolling movement smoothly, place your hands under your thighs. Focus on your abdominal contractions and "scoop" your lower abdomen to begin and end the roll.

Repetitions
Repeat the exercise five times.

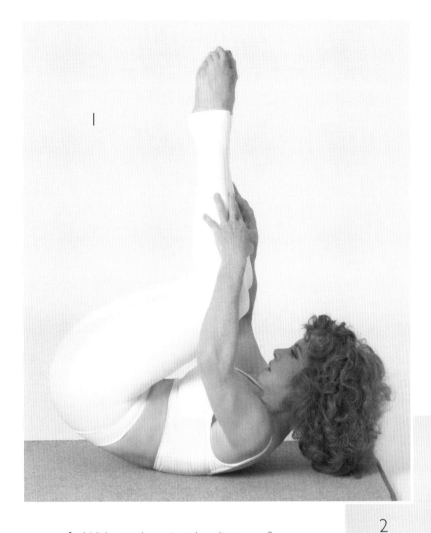

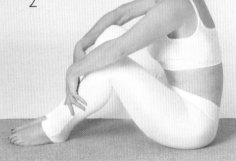

1 *Without changing the distance from your shoulders to your knees, roll back like a ball on to the mat. Roll slowly and with controlled precision, touching each vertebra to the mat. Roll only to your shoulder blades; never on to your neck.*

2 *Roll up to the sitting position, keeping your back rounded.*

Leg extensions

The first part of this exercise stretches the hamstrings in your legs while the second part is an abdominal challenge. The aim is to help your body achieve balance by maintaining an equilibrium between strength and flexibility. The core control necessary to perform the abdominal contraction while maintaining your alignment is the foundation of Pilates work.

Breathing pattern

• Inhale as you extend your legs.

• Exhale as you bend your knees.

• Repeat the inhale–exhale pattern as you progress to the larger V.

• Take a full breath as you extend your legs and prepare for the abdominal contraction.

• Inhale as you lengthen your spine.

• Exhale as you contract your abdominal muscles.

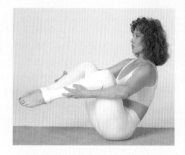

Starting position
Sit down, bend your knees to your chest, and hold on to your calves. Lift your legs off the mat and open your knees until they are shoulder-distance apart. Keep your feet together.

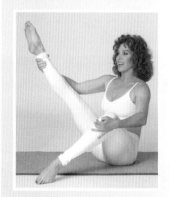

What you should feel
Your hamstrings and calf muscles will feel stretched and toned, and you should be able to feel your core strength and balance improve.

Variation
If you cannot fully extend your legs, do the exercise one leg at a time. If you roll over with your contraction, do the exercise with your feet on the floor.

Repetitions
Repeat both parts of the exercise four times.

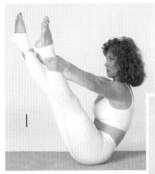

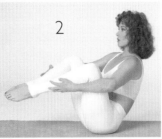

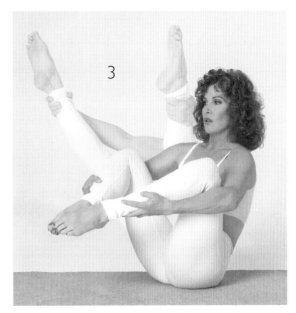

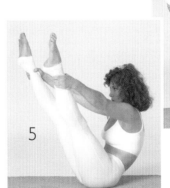

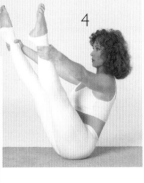

1 Extend your legs toward the ceiling to form a V position. Your legs should be shoulder-distance apart.

2 Bend your knees, keeping them at shoulder level. Bring your toes together but keep your feet off the mat.

3 Repeat this extension four times, with your legs extending wider with each repeat.

4 Extend your legs to the original V position. Lengthen your spine, stretching sequentially from your tailbone to the top of your head. Hold your legs still and straight.

5 Round your back and pull your lower abdominal muscles inward and upward. As you do so, stretch the small of your back and scoop your abdomen to curl your pelvis.

Do's and don'ts
* Keep your legs closer to your torso as you extend them. * Don't move your legs from your hips to your thighs. * Extend your legs only from your knees to your toes for the maximum stretch. * Keep pressing your shoulder blades down, away from your ears.

Open-leg rocker

The total coordination of your abdominal strength and spinal flexibility is put to the test here. Control is the key to the symmetry of this exercise. If you could not complete the last two exercises (see pp.86–9), do not attempt the open-leg rocker. This is because you will not be using the correct muscles to do the movement properly and you could put undue pressure on your back.

Throughout the exercise, keep your arms straight and never roll back further than your shoulder blades.

Breathing pattern

- Inhale as you roll back.

- Exhale as you roll up.

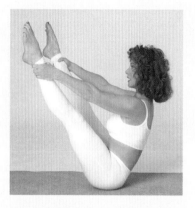

Starting position
Sit down, bend your knees to your chest, and hold on to your ankles. Lift your legs off the mat and open your knees until they are shoulder-distance apart. Keep your feet together, then extend your legs toward the ceiling to form a V position with your feet about shoulder-distance apart.

What you should feel
Your flexibility and control of movement will improve, and you should feel an increase in your abdominal strength.

Repetitions
Repeat the exercise five times.

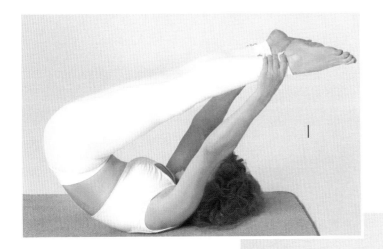

1 *Round your back and pull your lower abdominal muscles inward and upward, stretching the small of your back on to the floor and scooping your abdomen to curl your pelvis. Continue to round your torso, rolling back on to your shoulder blades.*

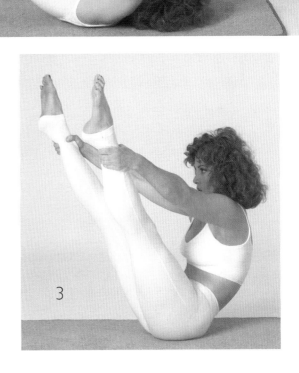

2 *Continue to roll back with your legs straight out from your hips, and bring them parallel to the floor over your head. Keep your head up and in line with your spine, so that it does not initiate the movement or touch the mat.*

3 *Roll up to your starting position and balance, with your abdominal muscles contracted and your pelvis curled under.*

Flex and point release

For a dynamic test of core strength and control, this exercise is a showstopper. It is more difficult than it looks and tests whether you are really using core strength or momentum. All the muscles in your pelvis are actively engaged to prevent any movement or change in your body design when you release your legs. Do this exercise after completing the open-leg rocker (see pp.90–1).

Breathing pattern

• Inhale as you flex your feet.

• Exhale as you point your feet.

• Take a full breath as you release your legs and hold them up.

• Take a full breath as you lower your legs to the floor.

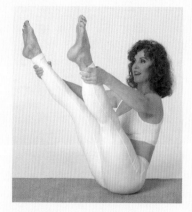

Starting position
Hold the open-leg rocker position, with your legs extended toward the ceiling in a V formation and your feet shoulder-distance apart.

What you should feel
Your flexibility and control of movement will improve, and you should feel an increase in your abdominal strength.

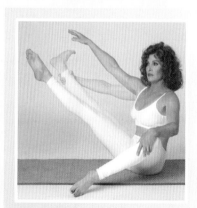

Variation
Work with one leg at a time, keeping your other leg bent.

Repetitions
Complete the sequence once only.

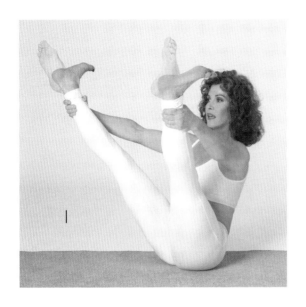

1 *Flex your feet and point your toes four times.*

2 *Let go of your legs and take a full breath before lowering your legs to the floor.*

3 *As they lower, stretch your arms upward and lengthen your spine.*

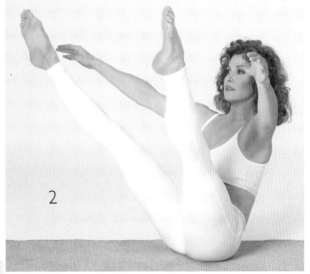

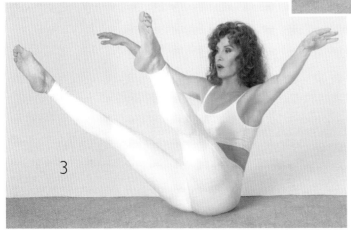

Do's and don'ts
* Make sure your torso stays rounded.
* Keep your shoulders directly over your hips.
* Don't lean back.
* Always achieve balance from core strength and focus.

Spine stretch

This exercise promotes good posture and spinal flexibility, coordinating hip stability with abdominal contraction. It is a navel-to-spine movement that teaches you how to connect all the muscles in the abdomen.

Breathing pattern

• Inhale as you sit tall and elongate your spine, opening your ribcage for a full expansion of your lungs.

• Exhale as you flex and contract, closing your ribcage in front of your torso with the strong abdominal contraction for a long, full exhalation.

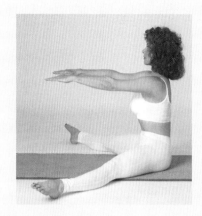

Starting position
Sit with your legs extended, then open them to a V position. Sit tall, stacking one vertebra on top of another. Press your shoulders down, away from your ears, and lift your arms in front at shoulder level.

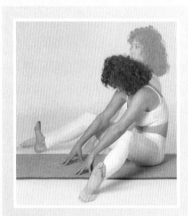

Variation
To begin the stretch, place your hands on the floor between your legs. Slightly soften your knees to reduce stress in your hamstrings.

What you should feel
The flexibility of your spine will increase, your hamstrings will feel elongated, and your abdominal muscles toned.

Repetitions
Repeat the exercise eight times.

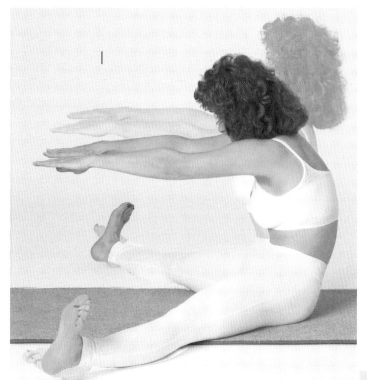

Do's and don'ts
* Anchor your feet strongly to the floor as you stretch and round your back.
* Stretch out your arms until they envelop your ears and your body forms a C shape.
* Let your spine grow long each time you release a contraction, then sit up out of your hips. * Don't let your knees rotate inward or outward as you stretch.

1 Point your toes and lengthen your spine, stretching the space from vertebra to vertebra. Flex your feet and contract your abdominal muscles, pulling from navel to spine and rounding your back.

2 Keep your shoulders over your hips and do not slump down. Imagine a thick band around your waist, 10cm (4in) above and below your navel. Pull your abdominal muscles inward and upward, as if someone is pulling the band directly behind your back. Your waist will not tip up or sink down, but stretch directly behind your back.

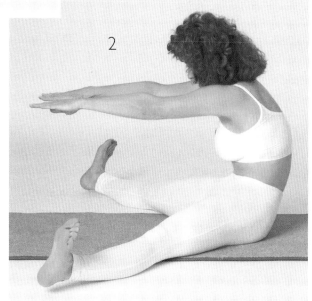

Twist

This exercise is more difficult than it seems, but if you practice it properly you can improve your symmetry by correcting imbalances between the two sides of your body. In order to work your body in balance you need to focus on individual aspects and the muscles involved. For example, the benefits come from elongating and rotating your spine, not by using your arms.

Breathing pattern

• Take two breaths as you twist your body to the side.

• Take two full breaths as you untwist your body to the center.

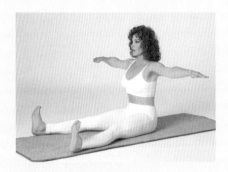

Starting position

Sit with your legs extended in front of you. Open your legs to the V position, slightly wider than your hips. Sit very tall, stacking one vertebra upon another. Press your shoulders down, away from your ears, and lift your arms out at shoulder level.

Do's and don'ts

* If one side is more mobile than the other, stretch your tight side first. * Anchor your hips evenly to the mat to increase your spinal rotation. * Keep your head in line with your spine so that it follows the twist of the movement. * Don't let either arm come in front of your body as you twist your torso, or you will lose your anchor point. * Use your breath to pace the exercise. * Don't rush the twist or the return to the center. * Don't forget to lift up and off your hips despite the fact that you are sitting on them – sit off from them instead.

What you should feel

Your waistline will feel toned and you will be able to rotate your spine more easily.

Repetitions

Repeat the whole exercise four times.

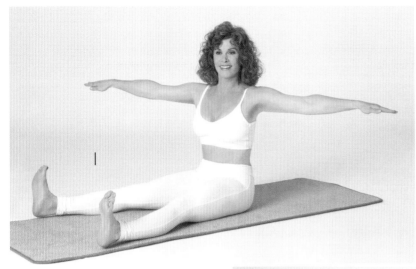

1 *Lengthen your spine, stretching the space between vertebrae. Twist to one side, elongating your back muscles and keeping your ribcage closed. Keep your arms straight out, at shoulder level.*

Turn your torso to face your leg in four movements, twisting a little more each time.

2 *Twist to the center with the same four movements.*

Repeat the exercise on the other side.

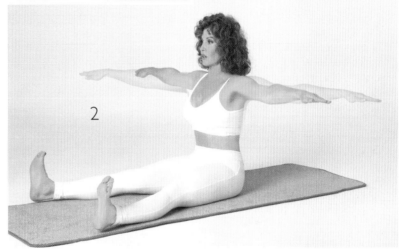

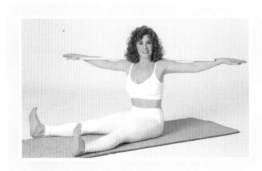

Variations
Before trying the twist, stretch your hamstrings with the spine stretch (see p.94) and do the towel exercises (see Chapter 3) to build up strength and increase flexibility.

Once you can do the twist easily, try doing it with a light pole or broomstick across your shoulders.

Twist with arm presses

This exercise will significantly benefit you if you play tennis or golf, as it stretches and strengthens the muscles around the spine. If you twist equally to both sides, lifting up and off from your hips and with an evenness of muscle strength and flexibility, you can balance the rotation of your spine.

Breathing pattern

• Inhale twice as you twist your body to the side.

• Do a double exhale and a double inhale for the pulses.

• Exhale twice as you untwist your body toward the center.

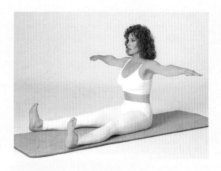

Starting position
Sit with your legs extended and open your legs to a V position, slightly wider than your hips. Lift your arms out at the sides at shoulder level. Flex your feet and lengthen the backs of your legs toward the mat.

Variation
If you feel any tension in your neck, press your shoulders down and back, and reduce the repetitions.

What you should feel
Any tension and stiffness in your back and neck muscles will be relieved. The exercise should also tone your upper arm muscles and improve your core strength.

Repetitions
Repeat the whole exercise four times.

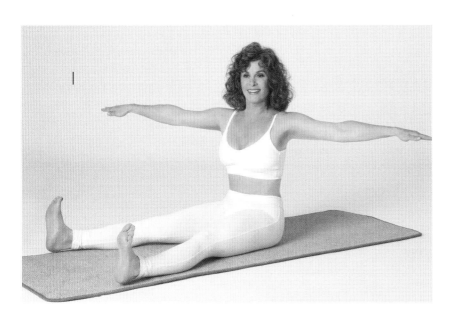

1 Lengthen your spine, sitting up out of your hips and stacking the vertebra on top of each other. Twist to one side, elongating your back muscles. Keep your ribcage closed and your arms directly out at shoulder level.

Turn your torso toward your leg in four movements, twisting a little more with each turn.

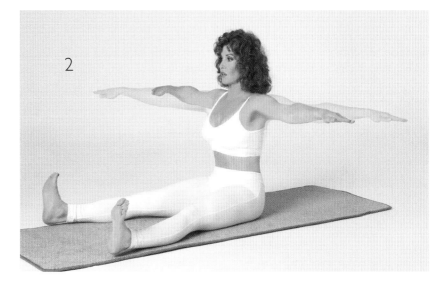

2 Twist to the center with the same four movements. Squeeze your shoulder blades together and pulse your arms back eight times.

Repeat the twist on your other side.

Saw

The saw works your waist and stretches your back muscles and hamstrings. If you do it with precision and concentration, it can be a perfect rotational stretch.

Breathing pattern

- Inhale and exhale, then turn your torso to the side.

- Inhale as you lift your arm. Exhale as you stretch over your leg.

- Inhale twice and exhale twice for each of the pulses.

- Inhale as you round your spine and exhale as you bring your arms out at shoulder level.

- Inhale and exhale after you rotate your torso to the center.

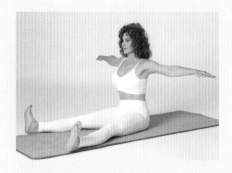

Starting position

Sit with your legs extended and open your legs to a V position, slightly wider than your hips. Lift your arms out at shoulder level and stretch them as if you are going to touch the walls on both sides of the room. Flex your feet and press your legs to the mat, all the way from your buttocks to your heels.

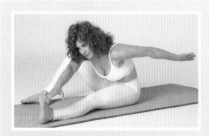

Variations

Soften your knees if you cannot sit up with your legs straight. Try bending one knee at a time, keeping the leg that you are stretching over straight.

For a more advanced version, try this exercise in a standing position, stretching over to the opposing foot on the floor.

What you should feel

Your spine will be more flexible, your legs and torso muscles stretched, and your lung capacity improved.

Repetitions

Repeat the whole exercise four times.

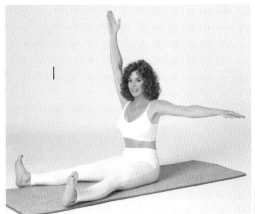

1 *Twist to the left side from your waist, keeping your ribcage closed, both hips evenly pressed to the mat, and your arms directly out at shoulder level. Lift your right arm up toward the ceiling.*

2 *Pull your abdominal muscles inward and upward, and stretch your left hand past the toes on your right leg. Stretch your right arm behind you. Keep your abdominal contraction and work in opposition, as if you have a thick band around your waist and someone is pulling it back behind you.*

Gently pulse forward eight times with a "sawing" motion.

3 *Round your back to sit up and lift your left hand toward the ceiling. Turn to the center, rotate your torso to the other side, and repeat Step 2.*

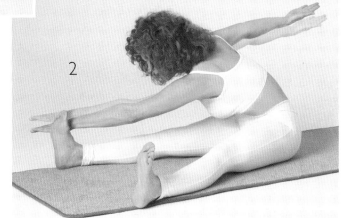

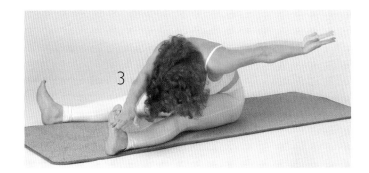

Do's and don'ts
* Make sure your head follows the line of your spine. * Stretch the top of your head toward your foot to avoid distorting your neck position. * Lift up and over your hips with a straight back. Don't curve over – feel the stretch from the hip joint.

Saw with arm presses

This exercise combines three difficult patterns and challenges the intricate muscular system of your core. All the powerhouse muscles benefit from keeping your spine erect and maintaining pelvic stability while rotating and pulsing. Make sure that you always sit up out of your hips and work in opposition.

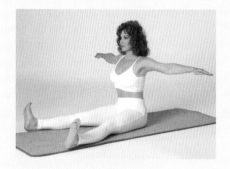

Breathing pattern

• Exhale twice as you twist to the side.

• Inhale as you lift your arm. Exhale as you stretch over your leg.

• Inhale twice and exhale twice for each of the pulses.

• Inhale as you round your spine and exhale as you bring your arms out at shoulder level.

• Do a double inhale and a double exhale for the arm pulses.

• Inhale twice as you untwist your torso toward the center.

Starting position

Sit with your legs extended, then open them to a V position, slightly wider than your hips. Lift your arms out at shoulder level. Flex your feet and lengthen the backs of your legs toward the mat.

What you should feel
Your upper arm muscles should feel toned, while your back muscles are balanced.

Variation
Complete each individual exercise before linking them in this pattern. If you begin to slump in your torso, only do one repetition on each side.

Repetitions
Repeat the whole exercise four times.

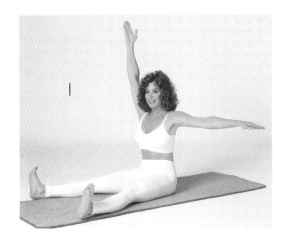

1 *Lengthen your spine, sitting up out of your hips and stacking the vertebra on top of one another. Twist to the left side, elongating your back muscles. Keep your ribcage closed and your arms directly out at shoulder level. Turn your torso toward your leg in four movements, twisting a little more each time. Lift your right arm toward the ceiling.*

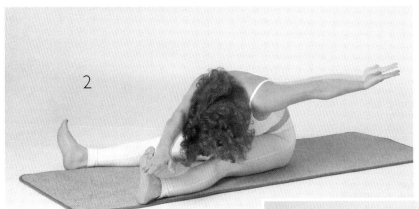

2 *Pull your abdominal muscles inward and upward. Stretch forward, reaching your right hand past the toes on your left foot.*

Pulse forward eight times as if "sawing" off your toes with the edge of your hand.

3 *Round your back to sit up, your torso still facing the same leg. Stretch your arms out at shoulder level.*

Squeeze your shoulder blades together and pulse your arms back behind you eight times. Keep your torso stable and don't move your chest or ribcage.

Twist to the center with four movements, then repeat the sequence on your other side.

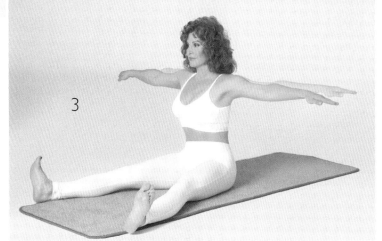

Circle in the sand

Each day we take for granted our ability to twist and turn until a stiff or strained muscle limits our normal movements. This easy twisting stretch keeps the body supple by working in a full circle around the body. Feel both hips anchored on the mat as you trace the largest circle you can.

Breathing pattern

• Inhale as you stretch your arm behind your body.

• Exhale as you circle your arm around the front of your body on the floor.

• Inhale as you lift your arm overhead and

sit up.

• Exhale as you lower your arm to the floor.

What you should feel
You should feel a greater release of the hip joints, greater flexibility in your waist, and your spine will feel elongated from vertebra to vertebra.

Repetitions
Repeat the exercise four times, alternating sides.

Starting position
Bring your feet together and bend your knees to form a diamond with your legs (see p.62). Sit tall and lengthen your spine upward.

Stretch one hand to the floor at the side of your body, with your arm straight and your fingers reaching away from your torso.

Variation
If your range of motion is restricted, stabilize your hips and contract your abdominal muscles as you twist back and stretch around.

For a more advanced movement, begin with eight pulses to the back and add eight more pulses as you stretch to your hand.

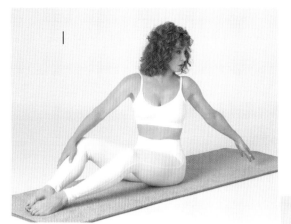

1 *Contract your abdominal muscles and reach your fingertips behind you as far as you can, keeping them on the floor. Keep your opposite shoulder and arm stable. Make a strong contraction, pulling your abdominal muscles inward and upward, and pulling your navel toward your spine.*

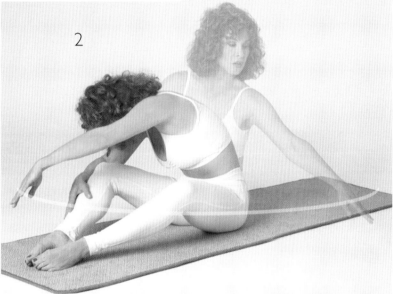

2 *Trace a circle on the floor with your hand as you curve your torso over your diamond and circle to the other side of your body. Do not stop until your arm comes all the way round to your other hand.*

3 *Lift your arm up toward the ceiling, rounding your torso up to a sitting position. Finally, lower your arm to the floor at the side of your body.*

105

Flat presses

This exercise may at first seem simple, but it works the body from the inside out to increase spinal alignment. Work with focus and concentration to feel the movement from the bones, not the muscles.

Breathing pattern

• Inhale twice as you press your lower back to the floor.

• Exhale twice as you release your lower back.

• Inhale twice as you press your shoulders to the floor.

• Exhale twice as you release your shoulders.

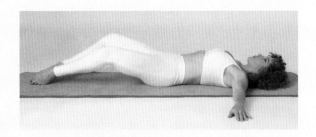

Starting position

Sit down, bring your feet together, and bend your knees to form a diamond with your legs. Contract your abdominal muscles and roll your spine to the mat, imprinting each vertebra. Extend your arms at shoulder level, with palms down. Relax the tension in your back and neck muscles.

What you should feel
As your spine sinks into the mat, all tension will gradually disappear.

Repetitions
Press your lower back and your shoulders to the floor, four times each. Repeat the exercise, alternating the press from your lower back to your shoulders.

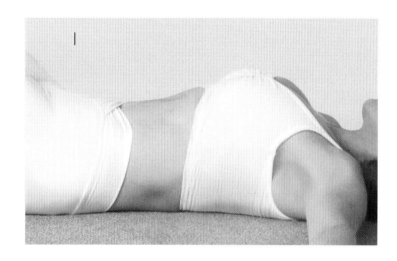

I *Press your lower back to the mat, without curling your pelvis. Release the press without tipping your hips or letting your back lift off the mat.*

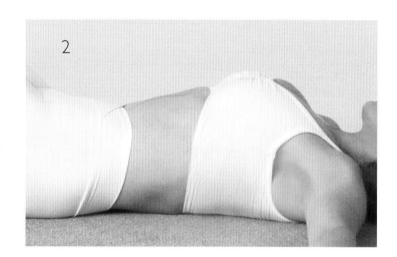

2 *Press your shoulders to the mat without allowing your ribcage to flare open.*

Release your shoulders, keeping your shoulder blades pulled down, away from your ears, and your neck relaxed.

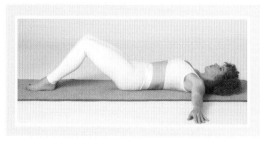

Variation
At first, your spine may not touch your mat at each vertebra. Overly developed curves and tight muscles will prevent you from allowing a complete release. Work with your knees bent and feet flat on the floor to help relieve lower back tension and tight muscles.

Knee twist

This stretch is great for hamstrings and for back and chest muscles. It rotates the spine and works the torso with a twisting motion that decompresses your spine.

Breathing pattern

- Breathe in and out in the starting position.

- Inhale once as you press your knees to the side.

- Exhale twice as you hold the stretch.

- Inhale twice as you return to center.

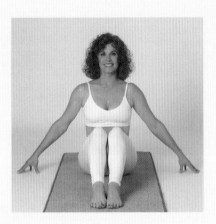

Starting position

Sit with your knees bent and your feet flat on the mat. Extend your arms to your sides and place the fingertips on the floor. Keep your arms straight and stretch your chest upward to prevent your shoulders from hunching forward. Your upper body needs to remain stationary through the entire exercise. Keep your knees together and point your toes, lifting your heels off the mat.

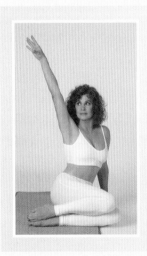

Variation
Once your legs are working together as a single unit, add an arm lift to the exercise. When your knees are pressed to the floor on the left side, keep your shoulders down and lift your right arm toward the ceiling. Place your hand on the floor and repeat the arm lift on the other side.

What you should feel
Your hamstrings and back and chest muscles will feel stretched and toned.

Repetitions
Repeat the whole exercise four times.

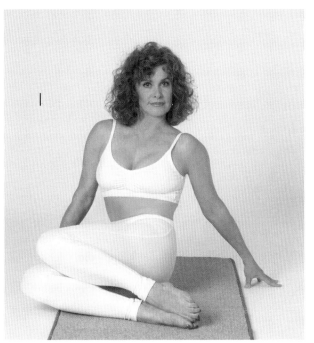

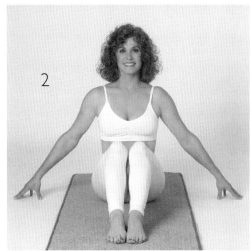

I *Press your knees to the floor to one side of your body. Keep them firmly together and pulse to the floor eight times.*

2 *Without letting them separate, lift your knees and return to the center position.*

3 *Press your knees to the floor on the other side of your body. Keep them together and pulse to the floor eight times.*

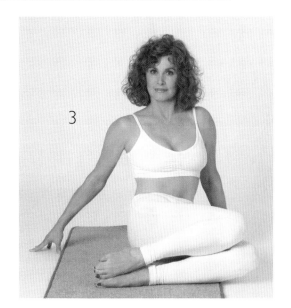

Do's and don'ts
* Press your shoulders down and back while lifting your chest up.
* Don't round your back. * Sit directly on your hip bones. * Scoop your abdominal muscles to resist the stretch by pulling your torso away from your legs. * Don't let your body weight lift off the floor.

Side stretch

This exercise builds upon the side stretch in Chapter 3 (see pp.50–1), where you decreased imbalances in your body by contracting the muscles on one side while lengthening the opposing muscle groups.

Breathing pattern

• Inhale and exhale as you lift and bend over your torso.

• Inhale twice and exhale twice as you pulse eight times.

• Inhale as you lift and exhale when you return to the starting position.

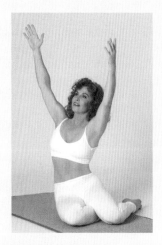

Starting position
Sit with your knees bent to the side of your body. Tuck your feet close to your hips, keeping both hips on the mat. Lift your arms up toward the ceiling.

What you should feel
The muscles in your upper body will feel strengthened and your waistline toned.

Do's and don'ts
* Keep your abdominal muscles contracted and your hips anchored for support. * Don't rest on your hips as you pulse – reach up and over the hips instead.

Repetitions
Repeat the sequence twice on one side, then twice on the other.

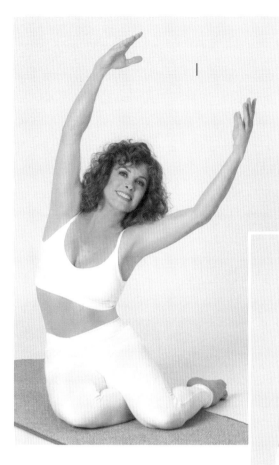

1 *Lift and stretch your torso to the side of your body, over your feet.*

2 *Pulse your arms eight times.*

3 *Twist into the center and return to the starting position.*

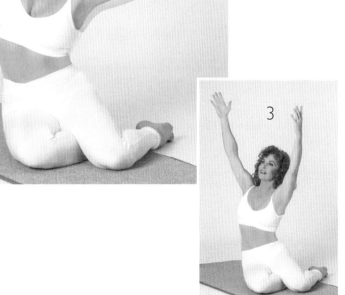

Single push-up

Push-ups focus on the muscles of the shoulders, upper back, chest, and arms. The unique position of the torso adds rotation to work the waist while decreasing any strain in the wrists and lower back muscles. This exercise moves smoothly and fluidly, concentrating on twisting and side bending for maximum waistline work.

Breathing pattern

- Inhale as you lift your arms.

- Exhale as you stretch over your feet.

- Inhale as you lower to the floor, placing your hands under your shoulders.

- Exhale as you lift your torso up.

- Inhale as you twist to the center position.

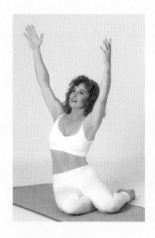

Starting position

Sit with your knees bent to one side. Tuck your feet close to your hips, keeping both hips on the mat. Stretch your torso to the side, over your feet. Lift your torso to the center, lift your hands over your head, and twist at the waist.

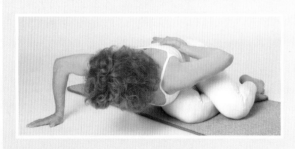

Variation

For a more advanced push-up, place one hand on the small of your back and complete the push-ups with a single arm. Focus on your alignment and feel the exercise in your upper back and arm muscles. Change hands and repeat.

Repetitions

Repeat the exercise eight times on one side, then eight times on the other.

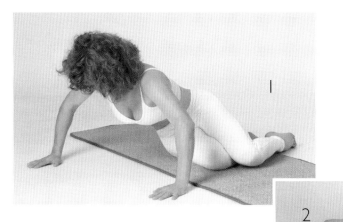

1

What you should feel
Your torso will be more flexible, your upper arms strengthened, your waistline toned, and you should feel increased strength and support in your upper chest.

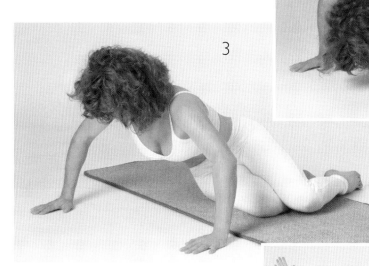

2

3

Do's and don'ts
* Keep your abdominal muscles contracted. * Keep a constant rhythm to the movements.
* Don't round your back – try to maintain a straight line.
* Keep your shoulders back and down, and your chest up. * Keep your elbows out and level.

4

1 *Contract your abdominal muscles and press both hips into the mat. Begin to lower your torso to the floor, placing your hands under your shoulders. Place equal weight into both arms and keep your shoulders level. Hold your back straight.*

2 *Bend your arms, bringing your elbows wide to the sides of your body and lowering your head so that your spine is parallel with the floor.*

3 *Push up, lifting your torso off the floor.*

4 *Twist back to the center position with your arms over your head.*

Side leg-kick series
– point up, flex down

The side leg-kick series of four exercises is specially designed to simultaneously stretch, tone, strengthen, and lengthen the leg muscles. Do these four exercises sequentially with one leg, before repeating them with the other. The first exercise – point up, flex down – emphasizes mobility and trunk stability, while lubricating the hip joint.

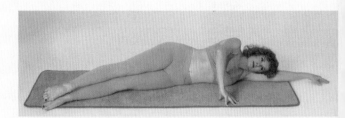

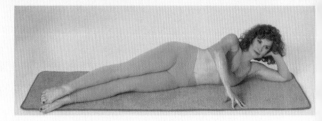

Breathing pattern

- Inhale twice as you lift your leg.

- Exhale twice as you lower your leg.

What you should feel
Your hips should feel more mobile, while your outer thigh muscles are toned.

Do's and don'ts
* Don't move your shoulders or hips. * Don't rock backward as you lift your leg. * Keep your knee facing forward. * Make sure the moving leg is long and straight.

Starting position
Lie on one side at the back edge of the mat. Form a straight line with your hips and back, placing shoulder over shoulder and hip over hip. Stretch your lower arm out on the floor and rest your head on it. With straight legs, bring your feet to the opposite edge of the mat at a slight angle.

If you wish, you may bend your lower arm and rest your head in your hand without distorting the alignment of your neck. Use your other hand in front of your chest for balance.

Repetitions
Repeat the sequence eight times.

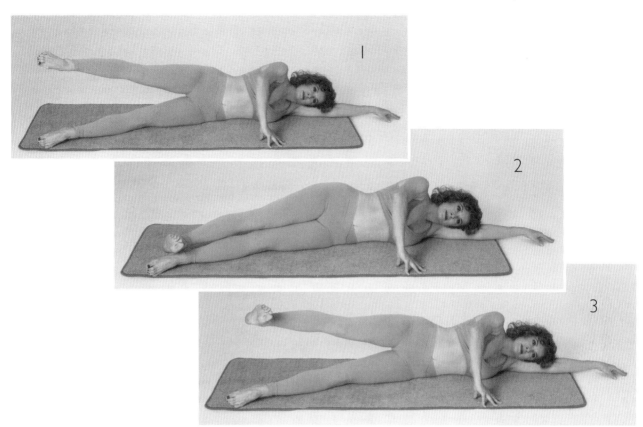

1 *Lift your top leg as high as you can, without rolling your hip or leg forward or back. Point the foot as you lift.*

2 *Lower the leg on top of the other leg, stretching it so that it reaches out of your hip and past your foot on the mat. Flex the foot as you lower the leg.*

3 *Repeat the exercise, but this time flex your foot as you lift the leg and point your foot as you lower it.*

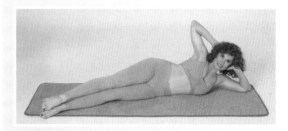

Variation
For a more challenging exercise, place your top arm behind your head with your elbow bent and pointing upward toward the ceiling. Let your fingertips touch, but don't clasp them together. The last exercise in the side leg-kick series (see pp.120–21) builds upon this variation.

Side leg-kick series – *pulse to sweep*

The most important aspect of this exercise is to use your core alignment to maintain the height of your leg as it sweeps forward and back. If it helps, visualize the space between your foot and the floor as solid so that your leg cannot go lower. If your hip rolls or releases, your leg will follow, causing uneven movement.

Breathing pattern

- Breathe in and out as you lift your leg.

- Inhale twice and exhale twice as you pulse your leg.

- Perform a long exhale as you sweep your leg backward.

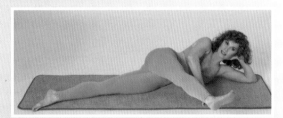

Variations

Use the alignment position that helps you to maintain your core stability. It is better to place your hand or head down on the floor for balance than to swing your leg around, releasing the solid positioning of your hips.

Flex your foot as you sweep it forward, and pulse and point your foot as you sweep it back. Then reverse the foot position – point it as you sweep it forward, and pulse and flex as you sweep it back.

What you should feel

Your core stability will improve while your leg muscles are toned.

Repetitions

Repeat the exercise eight times.

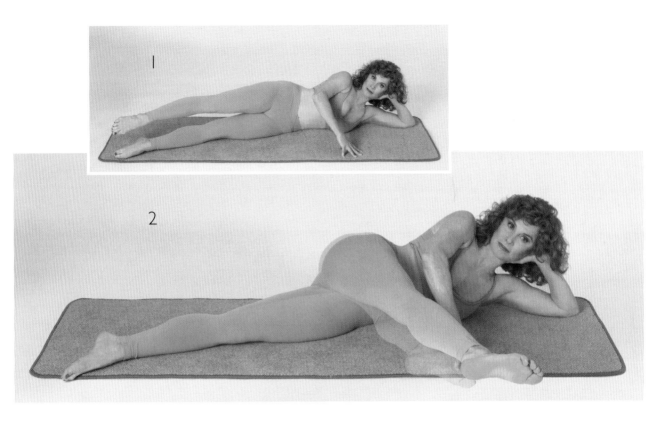

1 Lift your top leg until it is level with your hip and parallel to the floor. Stretch the space from your ribcage to your hip.

2 Sweep your leg forward without moving your hips or shoulders. Sweep only as far as you can without swaying.

Pulse your leg twice in front of your body.

3 Sweep your leg backward, keeping it hip-distance above the mat at all times.

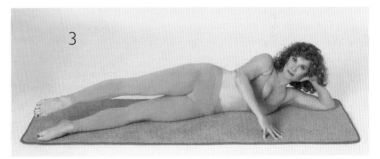

Do's and don'ts
* Maintain the support of the muscles in your abdomen and back. * Make sure you keep your hips and shoulders stacked. * Don't let your hip roll or release.

Side leg-kick series – *bicycle*

This exercise is like pedaling a bicycle with one leg. When your leg is bent in front of your body, the knee and foot should be the same distance from the floor. For correct trunk alignment, make sure you keep the top hip over the bottom hip, and top shoulder over the bottom shoulder.

As it becomes easier to combine all four side leg-kick exercises, the sequence will build crucial core resistance and strength.

Breathing pattern

- Take two full breaths to perform one cycle of the movement.

Variation
The advanced body position at Step 6 is very difficult to control. Work up to it slowly. Never sacrifice your body alignment for the sake of the movement. Until you gain enough core strength to sweep fully, keep the movement small. Keep your hand down on the mat for balance if your hips or shoulders move.

Repetitions
Do five movements pedaling forward and five pedaling back.

1 Bend your top knee in front of your body at hip level. Make sure it is parallel to the floor. Don't rotate your knee upward or downward.

2 Extend the leg in front of your body, stretching it out from hip to toes. Keep it at hip level.

3 Sweep your leg back as far as possible, maintaining your core stability and keeping your leg parallel to the floor. Hold the leg back, stretching from hip to toes.

4 Bend your leg in front of your body at hip level and parallel to the floor, as in Step 1.

5 Move your bent leg to the back of your body, then sweep it straight to the front of your body.

6 Bend your knee parallel in front of you, press your leg behind you, and then straighten your leg.

What you should feel
Your hip joint should feel more flexible, while your leg muscles are stretched and toned.

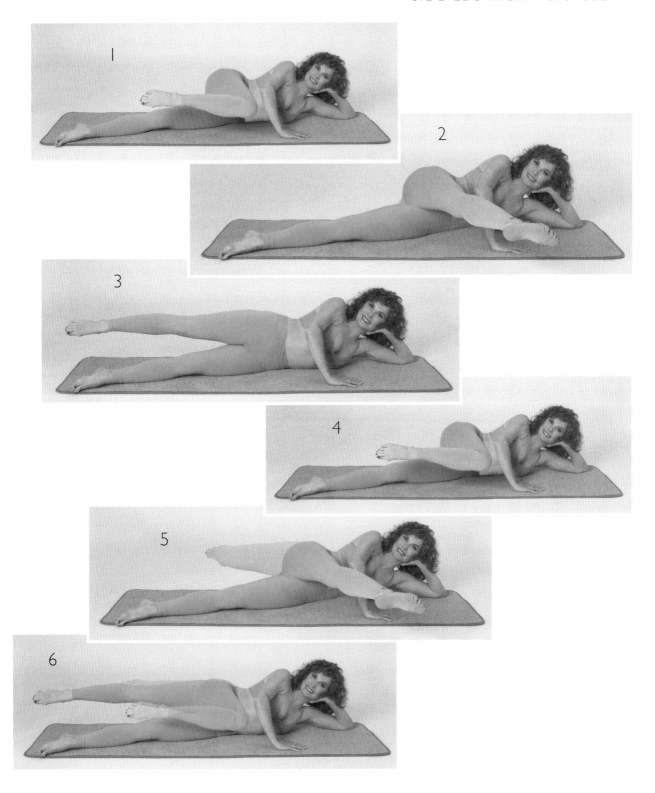

Side leg-kick series
– beats with point and flex

In this exercise, you need to stretch your leg longer with each beat so the movement is not pumping up and down, but extending past your bottom leg as you work. Use your breathing pattern to keep the rhythm of your movements. Do not attempt this advanced exercise until you feel strong enough to maintain the straight back and torso support.

Breathing pattern

• Inhale and exhale as you lift.

• Inhale twice and exhale twice as you beat the top leg.

1 *Lift your top leg as far as you can without twisting your knee upward or changing your hip alignment. Your knee cap must face forward. Keep your muscles elongated and both legs straight.*

2 *With the foot of the extended leg pointed, beat the top leg toward the floor with four small, sharp movements.*

3 *With the foot flexed, repeat the four beats.*

What you should feel
Your inner and outer thigh muscles should feel toned, while your core muscles are stretched.

Variation
To increase your lung capacity, gradually work up to four inhalations and four exhalations with each beat.

Repetitions
Alternate the point and flex movements and do four sets of each foot position.

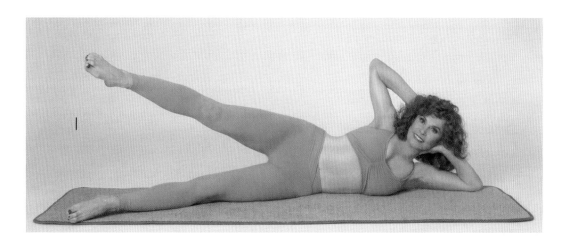

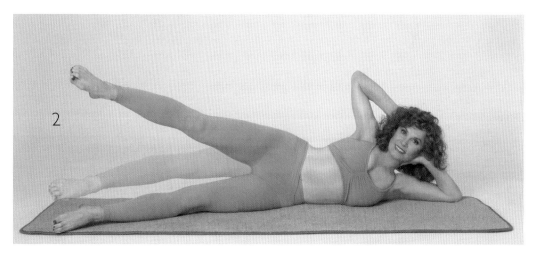

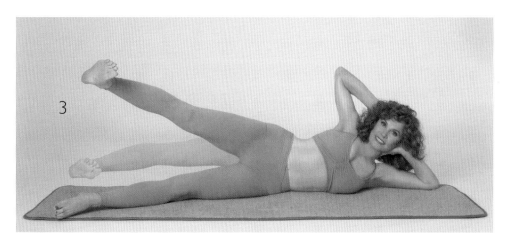

Roll-up to alignment

This exercise helps you to achieve proper muscular flexibility and to complete your workout by giving you a pattern that flows through your whole body.

Breathing pattern

- Inhale as you lift your heels and exhale as you lower them.

- Take full breaths as you circle your arms.

- Take two breaths as you roll up to standing.

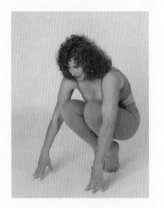

Starting position

Bring your feet and knees together. Roll on to the balls of your feet with your ankles together. Round your back and sit on your heels, placing your hands on the floor in front of your torso. Press your shoulders down, away from your ears, and relax your shoulders and back muscles.

Variation

Stand with your back against a wall with your feet 20–25cm (8–10in) from the base. With your shoulders pressed back into the wall and pulled down away from your ears, bring your chin to your chest. Roll one vertebra at a time, peeling your spine off the wall. Relax your arms. Keep your abdominal muscles contracted, your navel to your spine, and your tailbone pressed to the wall. Don't slump toward the floor, but visualize yourself rounding over a giant ball. Circle your arms in both directions. Roll slowly up the wall using your core muscles. Press the full length of your spine to the wall and breathe deeply.

Do's and don'ts

* Stack your vertebrae on top of one another as if you are pressing your spine into an imaginary wall. * Use your abdominal muscles and your powerhouse to control the exercise. * Work slowly and breathe deeply. * Don't forget to stretch through your neck bones so that the very last part to roll up is your head.

Repetitions

Complete the sequence once only.

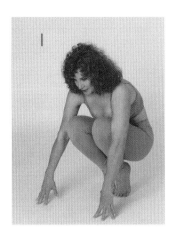

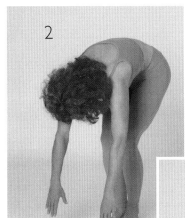

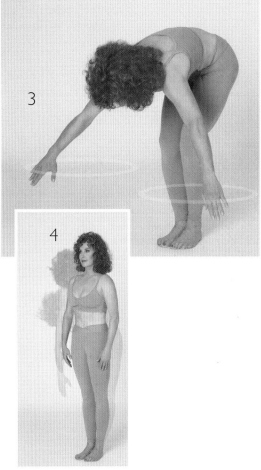

1 *With your heels lifted, roll higher on to the balls of your feet, staying centered on the front of your foot triangles. Lower your heels toward the floor, stretching your Achilles tendons and calf muscles. Repeat this movement eight times.*

2 *Slowly begin to straighten your legs, lowering your heels to the floor. Roll your body up to the point where your hands are off the floor. Pull your shoulders down, away from your ears, relaxing your neck muscles. Keep your knees bent and your back rounded. Pull your abdominal muscles inward and upward.*

3 *Slowly circle your arms. Circle eight times and make the circle larger with each repetition. Reverse and repeat the circles.*

4 *Continue to roll your torso up until you reach the standing position.*

What you should feel
Your spine will feel more flexible and your posture will improve.

Cool down

This exercise, which is a repeat of the core balance exercise (see pp.24–5), represents a final closing sequence. It will remind you how much the joints and muscles of your body have learned from practicing the Pilates technique. You can use it as a cool-down exercise to bring your Pilates practice to a close and you can also use this alignment to perform your daily tasks.

Breathing pattern

• Inhale as you lift your toes.

• Breathe deeply, inhaling and exhaling with your eyes closed.

• Inhale as you open your eyes. Exhale as you lower your toes.

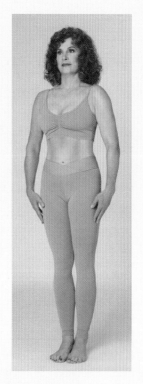

Starting position
Stand with your feet together. Align your body, finding your center. Tighten your hips and shoulders. Do not sway or arch your back or tuck your pelvis forward. Lengthen the space from the top of your hips to the bottom of your ribcage. Place your head directly on top of your spine.

What you should feel
Your balance will improve as your core alignment strengthens.

Repetitions
Repeat the exercise three times.

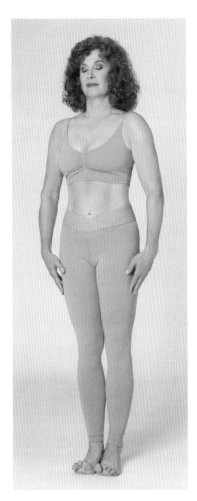

1 *Close your eyes. Inhale and exhale deeply. Then inhale as you lift your toes.*

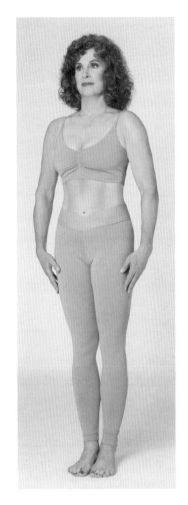

2 *Open your eyes and exhale as you lower your toes.*

Variations

Add another breath with your eyes closed and toes lifted, and work up to five breaths.

For ultimate balance control, lower your toes and lift one foot off the floor. Close your eyes and take a full breath. Open your eyes and lower the foot to the floor. Repeat with your other leg. Pay close attention to the different inner corrections that your body makes on each side. Your body imbalances are easier to recognize with your eyes closed. Use this tool to begin to balance your body from the inside out with the Pilates method.

6 Appendix

* **The seven elements**

* **Advanced breathing**

* **Body positions**

* **Actions**

* **The key muscle groups**

* **Planning your program**

* **Exercise programs**

This appendix is designed to help you develop and understand the Pilates technique as illustrated in this book. As you practice, try to remember the seven mind–body elements on the opposite page. The instructions on advanced breathing techniques will help you to improve the oxygenation of your body's cells. Refer to the sections on body positions and actions if you need to clarify a particular term used in the book. The anatomy page will help you to locate the position of some of the major muscle groups in the body. Finally, program charts will help you to plan your Pilates practice and to organize it into exercise sequences.

THE SEVEN ELEMENTS

A few movements, properly performed, are worth more than hundreds of mindless repetitions. Try to make sure that each and every exercise in your Pilates program includes each of the following elements:

Concentration – Aways be constantly aware of how you are doing what you are doing. Stay focused and pay attention to every part of your body. When your mind directs an action, your body will respond better and the results will be more immediate.

Control – Concentration leads to control. Taking charge of your body and how you move enables you to work to your maximum potential without strain or risk of injury.

Centering – Your torso is your body's strength center and the starting point for every movement. Centering focuses on abdominal control and improves balance, posture, and alignment. Centering balances the body's weight in all positions, including standing, sitting, and lying down.

Precision – Precise positioning and exact movement fine-tunes your muscular system. Precision incorporates more muscles into

activity for more balanced muscle work. It prevents you relying on momentum and swinging your body, which can lead to muscle fatigue and strain.

Flow of movement – Focus on a flowing motion that utilizes your muscles holistically and matches and enhances the flowing movements of life. Rigid, stiff movements are replaced with grace and ease.

Breathing – Breath energizes and revitalizes the body. Each exercise is fueled by our breath and coordinated to every movement pattern. As with the flow of motion, the Pilates technique contains a continuous flow of breathing that creates a rhythm for movement.

Harmony – Integrate the above elements into every exercise. Working from your center with concentration, control, and precision creates a flow of movement coordinated with breathing. The conscious combination of these elements promotes a sense of well-being. This harmony does not end when you finish your work-out, but is carried into your daily activities, refreshing your mind, invigorating your body, and uplifting your spirit.

Advanced breathing

Joseph Pilates wrote: "Breath is our first act of life, and our last". Breath fuels our cells and nourishes our bodies. It affects our activity on every level, from the simplest daily task to intense physical activity or emotional stress. Breath is vital to the mind–body connection.

Breathing has two parts: diaphragmatic and thoracic. When we inhale, the diaphragm contracts, creating a vacuum in the chest (thoracic) cavity and the lungs so that air rushes in. When we exhale, the diaphragm relaxes, pushing out the air. Thoracic breathing expands and contracts the small muscles of the ribcage, causing it to open and close with ease and fluidity.

Deep-core breathing

All too often, and particularly as we age, our lung capacity decreases and we breathe only with the upper part of our lungs. This shallow breathing means that cells receive less oxygen and less carbon dioxide is removed. Deep-core breathing increases lung capacity, improving the oxygen supply and removing toxins.

Deep-core breathing combines the diaphragmatic and thoracic parts, and allows you to match the movement of the Pilates exercises to the way you inhale and exhale. Lung capacity is increased by dividing the inhalations and exhalations into equal parts, bringing oxygen in and expelling the air in two, three, four, and five parts.

Diaphragmatic breathing exercise

Place your hands on your abdomen, just below the navel. Inhale deeply, then slowly exhale. Inhale again and, as you exhale through your mouth, contract your lower abdominal muscles. Feel your abdomen pull inward as the contraction pushes more air out of your lungs. Inhale once again and, as you contract your lower abdominal muscles, thoroughly and sharply exhale through your mouth with a "shushing" sound. This method of breathing makes every exhale an abdominal exercise and will help to tone and flatten your abdominal muscles.

Thoracic breathing exercise

Place your hands on your ribcage, with your fingers touching at the center of your chest. Inhale through your nose, allowing your chest to expand and watch your fingers stretch apart. Exhale through your mouth and feel your ribcage close inward as your fingers touch once again. This simple movement of expansion and contraction involves all the muscles in your chest, neck, and upper back.

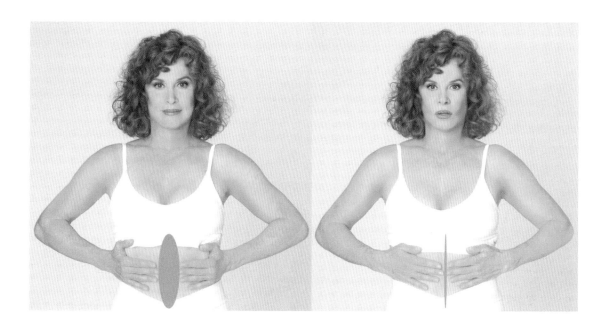

Deep-core breathing exercise

Place your hands on your ribcage, your fingers touching at the center. Inhale through your nose, expanding your chest. Watch the fingers stretch apart, noting the amount of space between them. Purse your lips together, make the "shushing" sound as you exhale. As your fingers come together, pull your lower abdominal muscles inward to fully expel the air from your lungs.

Divide the inhale into two parts, bringing in a greater amount of air. Exhale through your mouth in two parts with two "shushing" sounds. Repeat the exercise, dividing the inhales and exhales into three parts, then four parts, then five parts. Watch the space between your fingers grow as you increase the number of inhalations, expanding your chest and developing your lung capacity.

Practice this while you exercise for a few minutes a day. By the end of a month you will have advanced to a full program of exercise that will keep you fit and youthful.

BODY POSITIONS

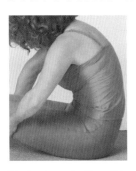

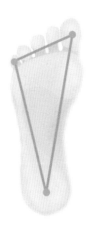

C shape – to form this position (above), contract your abdominal muscles inward as you release and stretch the back muscles. Reach the shoulders and hips slightly forward as you round the front of your trunk to form the letter C.

Foot centers or triangles – three foot centers on the sole (under the big toe, under the little toe, and at the center of the heel) form a triangle when connected (above). Focusing on the triangle will help you to distribute your weight evenly across the foot.

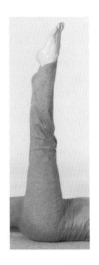

L position or 90 degrees – a right angle that is formed between your arms or legs and your trunk (above). The vertical reach is achieved by anchoring and stabilizing the torso while stretching the muscles of the extremities in opposition.

Keep the muscles pulling inward to prevent the opening or thrusting forward of the ribcage.

Shoulder positions – always gently reach your shoulders down and away from your ears. Proper placement involves stabilizing your shoulder girdles and the muscles underneath the shoulder blades, to prevent the shoulders from hunching, tensing, and lifting upward.

Spine (neutral) – a spinal position in which the back is neither tucked in nor arched. Instead, it is lengthened to activate the muscles in your core.

Tuck – the tilting or curling of the hips that flattens the lower section of your spine, tightening hip flexors and buttock muscles. Avoid tucking in your neutral or imprinted spine position.

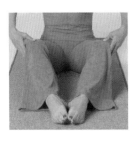

Diamond position – this is formed with your legs by bending your knees, opening your hips, and bringing the soles of your feet together (above). The diamond should be elongated so that your heels do not come too close to your pelvis.

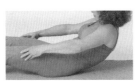

Imprint – as you roll down backward on to the mat, stretch and elongate your spine (above). This has the effect of pressing down one vertebra at a time and creating an "imprint" of your spine.

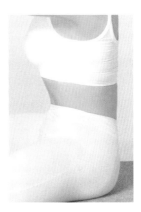

Ribcage placement – a technique in which you can lengthen the bottom of the ribcage away from the hip joints without releasing the muscles between the ribs (above).

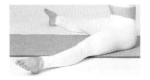

V position – a seated position in which your legs open to your sides, usually at a distance wider than your hips (above).

ACTIONS

Aligning your core – *your torso muscles are your core, or powerhouse. These include the shoulder girdle, chest, abdomen, back, and buttocks. Together, these muscles form your center of strength from which all movements are initiated. Aligning your core requires the awareness and use of all of these muscles.*

Anchoring – *anchoring is controlled mobility. By stabilizing your core, it produces greater stretch and muscle work. It allows you to move away from a fixed point in the body so that the muscles are activated to maximum potential.*

Contraction – *the activation or tightening of muscles without any strain or tension.*

Diaphragmatic breathing – *deep breathing that focuses on the conscious expansion and contraction of your diaphragm. It allows you to breath more deeply and to increase the volume of oxygen in your lungs.*

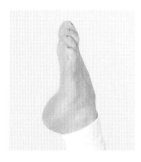

Extension – *movements that take your muscles, limbs, or trunk into a backward position – for example, the extension of the foot (above).*

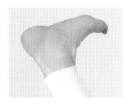

Flexion – *movements that take your muscles, limbs, and trunk into a forward position – for example, the flexion of the foot (above).*

Functional strength – *the ability of your body to perform movement as a holistic system in order to support daily activity, movement, and alignment.*

Navel-to-spine – *a Pilates term that refers to the initiation of the lower abdominal muscles. This is a contraction of the muscles from the top of the pelvis upward to the navel. When we say navel-to-spine, we do not just mean the "belly button", but the activation of all the muscles in the lower section of the abdomen.*

Opposition/opposing muscle groups – *for every action there is an equal and opposite reaction. As you contract or anchor one muscle group, the opposing muscle group will extend or lengthen.*

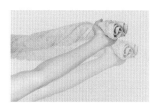

Pulse – *a movement that is small, controlled, and sustained – for example, a pulse of the arm (above). A pulse is initiated from a deep contraction.*

Range of motion – *the movement that is possible around a joint, such as the shoulder, or a set of joints. It involves the connecting muscles, ligaments, tendons, and bones.*

Release – *this term refers to a return to your starting position, not a "letting go" of the contracted muscles.*

Scoop – *a contraction that hollows the abdominal wall by pulling it flat and close to the spine. It does not involve the tuck of the pelvis or a change in shoulder alignment.*

Spinal articulation – *moving one vertebra at a time to stretch the bone from the disc, in order to increase the mobility of the spine and back. (See also Imprint, p.130.)*

Stabilization – *the maintenance of correct body alignment through movement. Stabilizing the joints allows the muscles to work to maximum benefit without risk of strain or injury.*

Thoracic breathing – *a component of breathing in which the ribcage is opened and closed at the front and back of the chest (thoracic) cavity.*

THE KEY MUSCLE GROUPS

Learning Pilates is like learning a new language for your body. These illustrations help you to locate the major muscle groups referred to in the book.

The torso or trunk (also known as the body's core) is not indicated, but is an area that extends across the shoulders, abdomen, and hips.

Spine
Cervical – the vertebrae in the neck.
Thoracic – the vertebrae that anchor the ribcage.
Lumbar – the vertebrae in the lower back, including the sacrum and coccyx.

Shoulder girdle *– the muscles surrounding the shoulder joint.*

Triceps *– three muscles at the back of the upper arm.*

Biceps *– two muscles at the front of the upper arm.*

Erector spinae *– the muscles that run vertically down the back, extending the spine and holding the body upright.*

Abdominals
(see below)

Abductor *– the muscles of the outer thigh, used for moving the leg outward.*

Hamstring *– the large muscle group at the back of the thigh.*

Quadriceps *– a group of four muscles located at the front of the thighs.*

Gluteus *– the maximus, minimus, and medius are the buttock muscles, the largest muscle group in the body.*

Hip flexor *– also known as the psoas muscle, it runs from the front of the leg to the hip joints.*

Achilles tendon *– the tendon at the back of the ankle used in flexion and extension of the foot.*

Abdominals
Internal and external obliques – the muscles used when rotating, bending, and extending the torso.
Rectus abdominus – the vertical muscles at the front of the abdomen, from ribcage to pelvis.
Transversus abdominus – the deepest of the lower abdominal muscles, it crosses the abdomen to the pelvic floor.

Adductor *– the muscles of the inner thigh, used in drawing the legs together or moving them inward.*

Planning your program

Life often gets in the way of exercise. Finding time in your hectic schedule to add any new program can be challenging, but with Pilates it will be worth it! You will increase your overall mobility and reduce muscle tightness and morning stiffness that steal valuable moments from your life. Use the following schedule as a guideline to gradually create an exercise routine that adds time to your day by increasing your physical aptitude and mental focus.

	Week 1	Week 2	Week 3	Week 4
Day 1	20-minute Stretch and Tone	20-minute Stretch and Tone	60-minute Full Program	60-minute Full Program
Day 2	10-minute Stretching	60-minute Full Program	20-minute Stretch and Tone	10-minute Stretching
Day 3	20-minute Stretch and Tone	10-minute Stretching	10-minute Stretching	60-minute Full Program
Day 4	10-minute Stretching	20-minute Stretch and Tone	60-minute Full Program	10-minute Stretching
Day 5	60-minute Full Program	60-minute Full Program	20-minute Stretch and Tone	60-minute Full Program
Day 6	10-minute Daily Maintenance	10-minute Daily Maintenance	10-minute Daily Maintenance	10-minute Stretching
Day 7	10-minute Stretching	10-minute Stretching	10-minute Stretching	60-minute Full Program

EXERCISE PROGRAMS

THE 10-MINUTE STRETCHING PROGRAM

Page	Exercise name	Muscle work
18	Single foot rolls	Increases flexibility of the muscles in the feet
24	Core balance	Improves balance; strengthens core alignment
26	Half circle and neck stretch	Stretches neck muscles; relieves stress and tension in neck and upper back
34	Towel lifts	Opens your shoulder girdle; builds upper body strength and shoulder joint flexibility
38	Towel pull-downs	Releases tension in the upper back; increases flexibility
50	Side stretch	Stretches and lengthens torso muscles; balances core muscles
56	Hip pulses	Stretches hip joints; strengthens the muscles at the sides of the hips
70	Hip lifts with circles	Lubricates hip joints; increases hip flexibility and tones inner and outer thigh muscles
86	Rolling like a ball	Increases spinal flexibility and develops strong abdominal muscles; improves breathing and circulation
94	Spine stretch	Increases spine flexibility; tones abdominal muscles
96	Twist	Tones the waistline; improves spinal rotation
104	Circle in the sand	Stretches waist and torso muscles; increases spine flexibility
108	Knee twist	Decompresses the spine; stretches back, chest and leg muscles
122	Roll up to alignment	Increases spinal flexibility; improves posture

THE 10-MINUTE DAILY MAINTENANCE PROGRAM

Page	Exercise name	Muscle work
20	Foot rolls with press	Stretches and strengthens the foot muscles
24	Core balance	Improves balance; strengthens core alignment
30	Finger flicks	Strengthens the muscles in the hands and forearms; improves circulation into the fingers
28	Cross foot stretch	Stretches and tones the muscles at the sides of the torso; improves balance
36	Taut pulls	Improves upper body strength; increases core alignment
40	Chest pull backs	Strengthens the muscles in the back and chest; works in conjunction with core strength to build a strong upper body
42	Overhead presses	Increases the mobility of the shoulder girdle; stretches the back, chest, and upper torso
52	Side stretch with arm reach	Stretches and lengthens the muscles of the torso; trims the waist
60	The Hundred	Improves breathing; stabilizes the trunk muscles and tones the abdominal muscles
72	Single leg pull	Tones the legs and abdominal muscles; stretches leg and back muscles
74	Single-leg side stretch	Stretches and tones hips and legs; increases core strength and alignment
102	Saw with arm presses	Balances back muscles; tones the muscles in the upper arms
106	Flat presses	Increases alignment in the shoulder girdle and hip joints; releases tension in the back muscles
122	Roll up to alignment	Increases spinal flexibility; improves posture

THE 20-MINUTE STRETCH AND TONE PROGRAM

Page	Exercise name	Muscle work
18	Single foot rolls	Increases flexibility of the muscles in the feet
22	Toe lifts	Stretches and tones the muscles on the top of the feet; improves circulation
24	Core balance	Improves balance; strengthens core alignment
28	Cross foot stretch	Stretches and tones the muscles at the sides of the torso; improves balance
34	Towel lifts	Opens the shoulder girdle; builds upper body strength and shoulder joint flexibility
38	Towel pull-downs	Releases tension in the upper back; increases flexibility
44	Behind the back stretch and lift	Balances the upper body strength and flexibility; relieves tension
46	Small presses up	Opens the chest to improve lung capacity; increases upper back and chest mobility
52	Side stretch with arm reach	Stretches and lengthens the torso muscles; trims the muscles at the waist
54	Overhead twist	Increases spinal flexibility; improves posture
62	Diamond to roll-up	Strengthens and flattens the abdomen; increase flexibility of the spine
64	Roll-up to diamond	Improves abdominal strength; increases the suppleness of the spine and back muscles
68	Traditional roll-up	Increases spinal flexion; strengthens abdominal muscles and stretches the back muscles
70	Hip lifts with circles	Lubricates the hip joints; increases hip flexibility and tones inner and outer thigh muscles
76	Double leg pull	Improves core spinal stability; tones abdominal and leg muscles
78	Double-leg side stretch	Increases flexibility of the hips; tones the legs and stretches the torso
86	Rolling like a ball	Increases spinal flexibility and develops strong abdominal muscles; improves breathing and circulation
88	Leg extensions	Improves core strength and balance; stretches hamstrings and calf muscles

110	Side stretch	Strengthens upper arm, chest and back muscles; tones the waistline
112	Single push-up	Tones the waistline; increases torso flexibility
114	Side leg kick series – Point up, flex down	Lubricates the hips; tones outer thigh muscles
116	Side leg kick series – Pulse to sweep	Tones leg muscles; improves core stability
120	Side leg kick series – Beats with point and flex	Improves muscles tone for the inner and outer thigh muscles; works core muscles
122	Roll-up to alignment	Increases spinal flexibility; improves posture

THE 60-MINUTE FULL PROGRAM

Page	Exercise name	Muscle work
18	Single foot rolls	Increases flexibility of the muscles in the feet
20	Foot rolls with press	Stretches and strengthens the foot muscles
22	Toe lifts	Stretches and tones the muscles on the top of the feet; improves circulation
24	Core balance	Improves balance; strengthens core alignment
26	Half circle and neck stretch	Stretches the neck muscles; relieves stress and tension in the neck and upper back
30	Finger flicks	Strengthens the muscles in the hands and forearms; improves circulation into the fingers
28	Cross foot stretch	Stretches and tones the muscles at the sides of the torso; improves balance
34	Towel lifts	Opens the shoulder girdle; builds upper body strength and shoulder joint flexibility
36	Taut pulls	Improves upper body strength; increases core alignment
38	Towel pull-downs	Releases tension in the upper back; increases flexibility
40	Chest pull-backs	Strengthens the muscles in the back and chest; works in conjunction with core strength to build a strong upper body
42	Overhead presses	Increases the mobility of your shoulder girdle; stretches the back, chest, and upper torso

APPENDIX

Page	Exercise name	Muscle work
44	Behind the back stretch and lift	Balances the upper body strength and flexibility; relieves tension
46	Small presses up	Opens the chest to improve lung capacity; increases upper back and chest mobility
48	Straight arm, back, and chest stretch	Lubricates shoulder joints; eliminates stress in the shoulders
56	Side stretch	Stretches and lengthens the torso muscles; balances core muscles
52	Side stretch with arm reach	Stretches and lengthens the torso muscles; trims the muscles at the waist
54	Overhead twist	Increases spinal flexibility; improves posture
56	Hip pulses	Stretches the hip joints; strengthens the muscles at the sides of the hips
60	The Hundred	Improves breathing; stabilizes the trunk muscles and tones the abdominal muscles
62	Diamond to roll-up	Strengthens and flattens the abdomen; increase flexibility of the spine
64	Roll-up to diamond	Improves abdominal strength; increases the suppleness of the spine and back muscles;
66	Diamond and spine roll	Tones and flattens abdominal muscles; increases core stabilization
68	Traditional roll-up	Increases spinal flexion; strengthens abdominal muscles and stretches your back muscles
70	Hip lifts with circles	Lubricates the hip joints; increases hip flexibility and tones inner and outer thigh muscles
72	Single leg pull	Tones the legs and abdominal muscles; stretches leg and back muscles
74	Single-leg side stretch	Stretches and tones hips and legs; increases core strength and a allignment
76	Double leg pull	Improves core spinal stability; tones abdominal and leg muscles
78	Double-leg side stretch	Increases flexibility of the hips; tones the legs and stretches the torso
80	Straight leg pull	Stretches and tones the legs and flattens the abdomen; stretches the hip flexors

Page	Exercise name	Muscle work
82	Leg stretch with arm reach	Increases flexibility of the hips and torso; tones the legs and stretches the arms and back muscles
86	Rolling like a ball	Increases spinal flexibility and develops strong abdominal muscles; improves breathing and circulation
88	Leg extensions	Improves core strength and balance; stretches hamstrings and calf muscles
90	Open-leg rocker	Increases abdominal strength and control of movement; improves flexibility
94	Spine stretch	Increases spine flexibility; tones abdominal muscles
96	Twist	Tones the waistline; improves spinal rotation
98	Twist with arm presses	Improves core strength; tones upper arm muscles
100	Saw	Increases spinal flexibility; stretches legs and torso muscles
102	Saw with arm presses	Balances back muscles; tones the muscles in the upper arms
104	Circle in the sand	Stretches waist and torso muscles; increases spine flexibility
106	Flat presses	Increases alignment in the shoulder girdle and hip joints; releases tension in the back muscles
108	Knee twist	Decompresses the spine; stretches back, chest and leg muscles
110	Side stretch	Strengthens upper arm, chest, and back muscles; tones the waistline
112	Single push-up	Tones the waistline; increases torso flexibility
114	Side leg kick series – Point up, flex down	Lubricates the hips; tones outer thigh muscles
116	Side leg kick series – Pulse to sweep	Tones leg muscles; improves core stability
118	Side leg kick series – Bicycle	Improves hip joint flexibility; stretches and tones leg muscles
120	Side leg kick series – Beats with point and flex	Improves muscles tone for the inner and outer thigh muscles; works core muscles
122	Roll-up to alignment	Increases spinal flexibility; improves posture
124	Cool down	Improves balance; strengthens core alignment

Index